Butterflies and Bananas

Blending Nature and Nutrition for Great Food and Family Fun

"Eat smart, stay fit, and walk gently with the creatures."

Blending Nature and Nutrition for Great Food and Family Fun

"Eat smart, stay fit, and walk gently with the creatures."

Marilyn Robinowitz

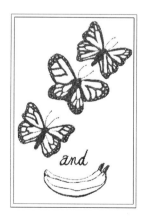

Contact information for Raul Gonzalez:
Raul Gonzalez rrgbuzz@gmail.com

First published by Dog Ear Publishing
4010 W. 86th Street, Ste H
Indianapolis, IN 46268
www.dogearpublishing.net

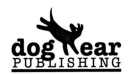

ISBN: 978-1-4575-2446-2

This book is printed on acid-free paper.

Printed in the United States of America

This book is dedicated to my grandchildren

Jared, Lilliana, and Camila

who motivate and inspire me.

The most important thing you can do for

your family is be a role model.

Embrace wellness!

Embrace life!

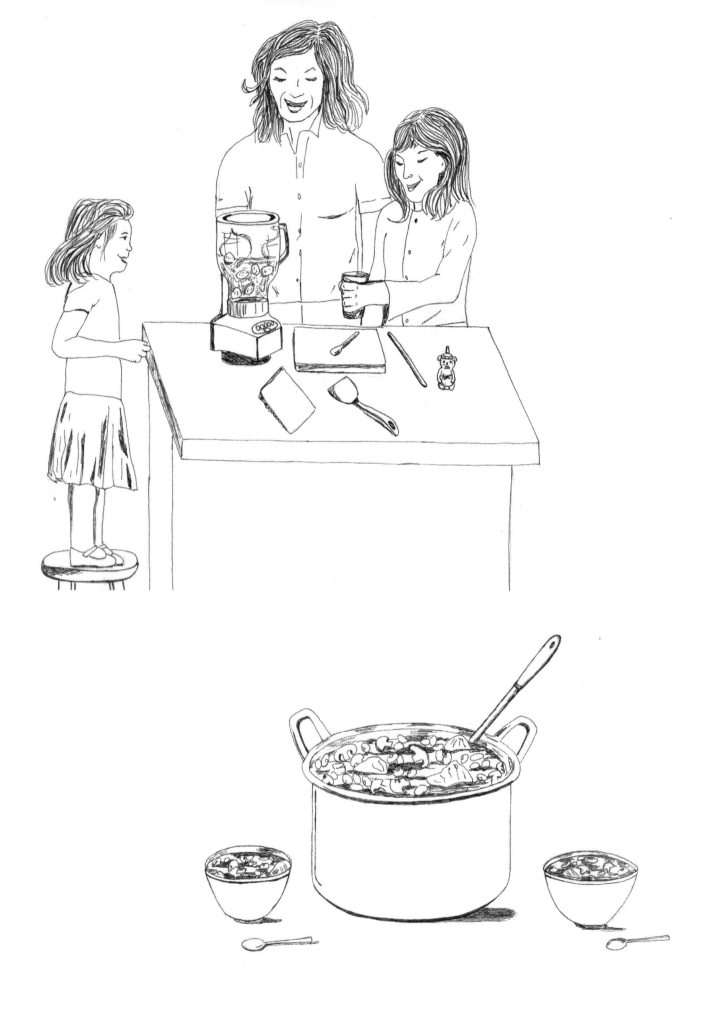

What This Book Offers You and Your Child

Exceptional Healthy Food

Nature Fascination

Family Fun

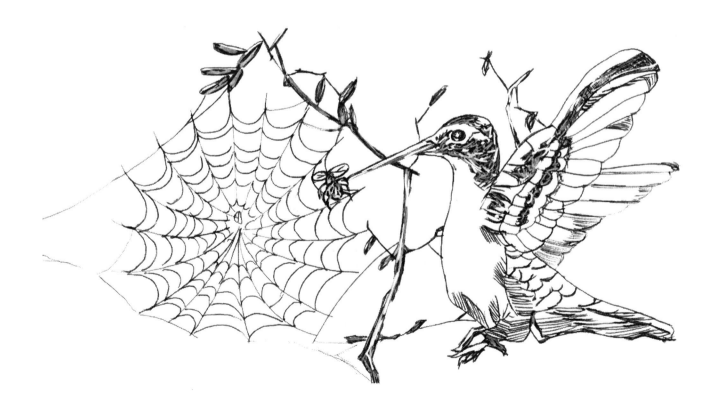

Contents

Chapter 4 - Make a Shake

Chapter 5 - It's a Green Thing

Chapter 6 - For the Love of It

*T*his book was a long time coming. Along the way to the publisher something wonderful happened: I grew, the book grew, and my grandson grew. I was also blessed with a lovely daughter-in-law who gave me, along with my son, two adorable granddaughters—now three and five—who inspire me every day to share my passions and do the things that I love. What have I learned from all of this? Never underestimate God's timing!

Of course, we all know 'life is not a bowl of cherries.' I have come to regard it as 'bittersweet.' You see, during the period of my writing I was faced with an aggressive form of breast cancer which required a year of treatment. The worst day of my life occurred when into three weeks of chemotherapy, I learned that my 51-year-old daughter—fit and exuberant as a young woman athlete—had suffered a stroke. Together, we held strong and every day I thank God for my daughter's strength, fortitude, and amazing courage through this difficult period.

As for me, my journey with cancer proved to be exactly as the young radiologist at M.D. Anderson Cancer Center said, "When all of this is over, you will be writing another chapter in your book and looking back at this as just a blip in your life." I said to myself, "Some blip!"

My daughter's health and vibrancy has also been restored. Is there a lesson here? I believe so. A fit body is a tremendous asset for anyone to own while recuperating from any surgery, illness, injury, or emotional trauma.

To have arrived at the place where I am today is the result of my own fortitude, and the two amazing institutions that boosted it: The Trotter Family YMCA in Houston, that first and foremost turned me into a physically fit person (I promise not to brag about my BMI); and the Houston Arboretum & Nature Center where my interpretive skills were honed. As a naturalist and school tour guide, I quickly learned that the voyage of discovery is as important as the interpretation. Are we not all hard-wired to want physical contact with nature?

Though I kept my writing well under cover for the first two years, I drew energy from many people, some who I am sure have not the slightest inkling of the role they played here. To those, I can only say, "Thank you. I am very grateful that you came my way."

The cast of characters in the making of this book is large, but had it not been for my husband and partner of sixty years, this book would not have been written. In good disposition, Rock critiqued every page that I wrote, even though I hogged the computer we shared.

We have always been a very functional family, but my children's assistance was above and beyond. They sensed when I needed help and came to my rescue. Both Robin and Bob participated in the editing, and it didn't seem to matter how busy they were.

My writing of this book did not come easy. I did it because I wanted to help create and share healthy and delicious food. My signature recipe, "One's a Meal Muffins," dates back to the 1980s, when oat bran was discovered as a heart healthy food and my interest in nutrition took hold. Today, Michael Pollan is my hero, and *Food Rules: An Eater's Manual* is my favorite book on food.

I am grateful to Ann Dodson, my favorite chef and caterer, who tested every recipe found in this book, which she did out of love. Her stamp of approval, corrections and suggestions made me feel confident and secure. I simply can't thank her enough. I have also been encouraged by the many family members and friends who have sampled and relished my food.

But what made the book come alive are the charming illustrations by Texas artist Raul Gonzalez. All of the illustrations are the result of a collaborative effort between the artist and the writer. Raul captured my vision and essence of the book. Raul is currently working on his Master of Fine Arts degree at The University of Texas, San Antonio, where 20 pieces of his artwork have been added to their permanent collection.

I am indebted to Pat Marks, associate director and head naturalist of the Houston Arboretum & Nature Center, who reviewed both Stump the Naturalist games in Chapter 5. Many thanks to Deborah Markey, our dynamic director at the Center, and again to Pat, for their permission to use the Scavenger Hunt Checklist and party theme. This activity has always been one of my favorites at the arboretum, and I am thrilled to include it in Chapter 5.

Many thanks to Jenny Garrett, formerly staff naturalist at the Houston Arboretum, who though incredibly busy at the time, graciously came by one day to read and assess some of my work in Chapter 4. I miss you, Jenny!

I also wish to thank the Oster family for participating in the Stump the Naturalist games, not once, but twice. The twice led me to create Part 2.

With her meticulous work on my notes and citations, Kate Brennan of Wits saved me lots of anguish and time. Thank you, Kate! Without your help and expertise it could not have been done.

And let it be known that Liliana Aguilar, nutritionist/dietician for the Trotter Family YMCA made a house call, and patiently checked all of the nutritional information and recipes in my book. Now Liliana, you can make the muffins you so much enjoyed, but please don't stop there.

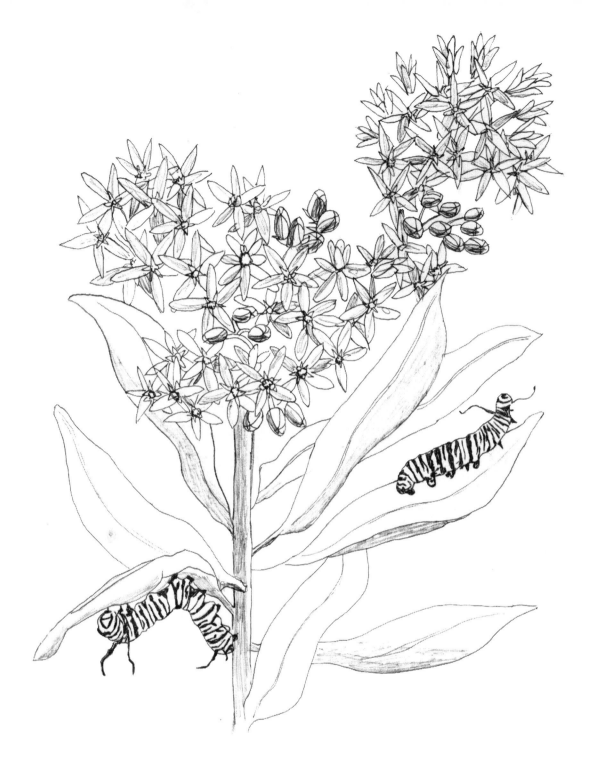

"For if one link in nature's chain might be lost, another might be lost, until the whole of things will vanish by piecemeal."

—Thomas Jefferson

Introduction

It was during my grandson's spring break from school that I began my love affair with shakes. He was nine years old. Every morning as I looked at the day's itinerary left for me by his mother, there would be this reminder: "Give Jared a healthy snack in the afternoon."

I met my daughter's request. I wanted the snack to be light and delicious. I decided to put some fruit, about to become overripe, in the freezer. The next day, an hour before baseball practice, I whipped up a strawberry shake using one percent milk for the protein, banana and strawberries for the carbohydrates, and a dash of honey for my grandson's sweet tooth. He loved it! Soon he was making shakes himself, adding his own signature with the addition of vanilla. It was fun. We made them often, using whatever fruit was available. When I returned home from visiting my grandson, the idea for a book was born.

This book is not about dieting. It is about awareness, mindful eating, and exercise; a lifestyle that eliminates the stress that comes with constant dieting, and instead promotes optimal health and a sense of well-being. With the right attitude, healthy eating and exercise can be fulfilling and fun.

When we educate ourselves, we come to regard food in the proper perspective. It was Benjamin Franklin who said, "Eat to live, and not live to eat; to lengthen thy life, lessen thy meals." I am sure if Franklin were alive today, he would agree that the ticket to good health in the 21st century is being physically active, eating a variety of the right foods, and knowing your portion size.

Just like adults, today's children have many demands to meet, and it is up to us as parents, grandparents, or caregivers to help them get what their growing bodies need and deserve.

This means the right food at the appropriate times; nourishment that will enable them to feel energized, motivated, and alert. In this book there are 18 delicious shake recipes (see Forest Index - page 25) that you and your children can enjoy as a snack or light meal.

Each shake will make one to two servings. The five dessert shakes are richer, but can be enjoyed on occasion as a treat. All are nutrient dense, supplying the body with healthy carbohydrates, proteins, and fats, along with the essential fiber often lacking in a child's diet. Combining our food in this way results in an even blood sugar response and energy that is maintained over a longer period of time.

The calories in these shakes are from whole foods, replacing calories found in junk foods. The body is replenished with vitamins and minerals that play an important role in combating disease. What's more, these shakes are a great way for children to get plenty of calcium, critical for the development of strong bones.

When we are physically active and eat right, we feel better; we are more aware—clued into our environment. We clearly see that all things in nature are inter-related; that an impact in just one of those things could have an effect, and then be felt all over. So while we work at getting our bodies healthy, let us also work at sowing healthy seeds—seeds that future generations will be harvesting. I call this "Eco-Fitness!"

Since our creatures hold such an important role in this equation, I have named each shake in my book after an animal, insect or bird. You will discover how beneficial these creatures are to the environment and to us. This diversion from the material world, in combination with these wholesome and delicious recipes, presents an exciting fun-filled opportunity for children, parents and caregivers to come together and explore. Healthy planet—healthy body!

As a naturalist, I am witness to children bonding with nature at a young age. I see firsthand the excitement and wonder on their faces as they explore the forest, ponds, and meadow habitats. Authentic nature fascination can happen if you follow the instructions in the chapter, "It's a Green Thing." Here you will find two creative and inexpensive birthday parties that will enable children and their chaperones to interact with nature firsthand. Evidence has shown that direct contact with nature is vital to the emotional and physical health of our youth.

In Chapter 6, "Recipes for Vibrant Living," I have included a collection of my favorite non-shake recipes that you and your family will enjoy making. They were created through the years for my family with the same love and passion that prompted me to write this book. They, too, are wholesome, delicious, and simple to prepare.

I am in awe of all parents do today, yet aware that many simply do not have the time or resources to plan and prepare healthy snacks and meals. With this is mind, all of my recipes in this book follow three guidelines:

> 1 - They must be easy to make and economical.
> 2 - They must be healthy and delicious.
> 3 - All ingredients must be available at most supermarkets.

I encourage you to invite your children into the kitchen to help whenever you are cooking, and to have at least one meal together every day. Besides, we all know that food is often equated with love, and who couldn't use an extra dose of that?

You can make this happen. Just begin by browsing through the entire book—connecting with the contents, index and illustrations. And when you return from the market with your bundle of nature's goodness, you know that you are on the right path to vibrant living.

Be aware—eat smart, stay fit, and walk gently with the creatures.

—Marilyn Robinowitz

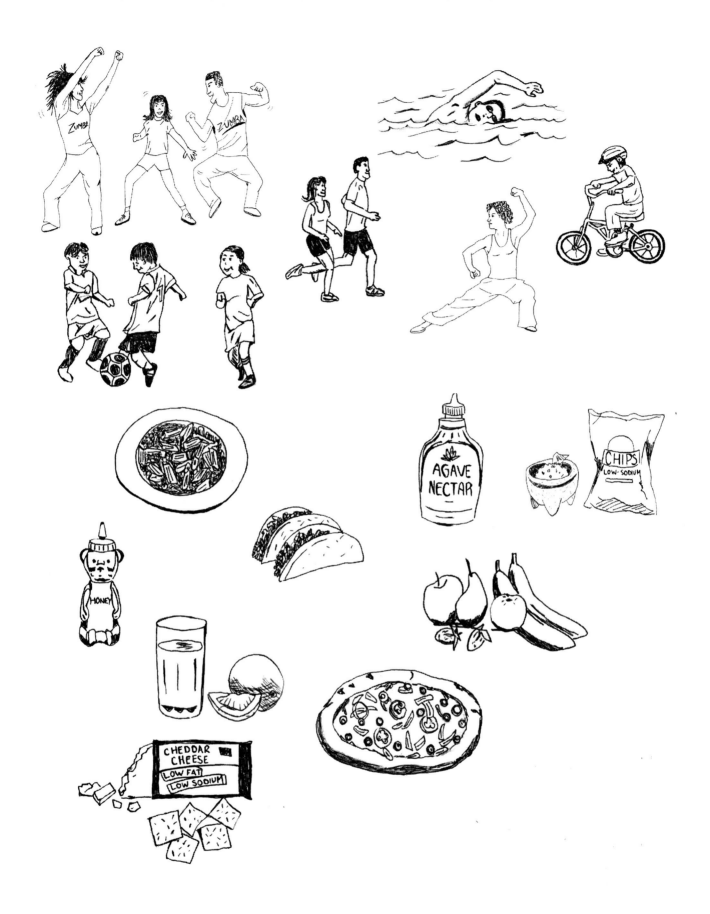

Find your balance   **Know your limit**

CHAPTER 1

What You Need to Know

Discretionary Calories

Why Physical Activity is Important

Good Ingredients

A Sweet Tooth

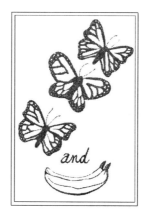

Discretionary Calories

What are discretionary calories? You need a certain number of calories to keep your body functioning and provide energy for your physical activities. Think of the calories you need for energy like budgeting money. Each person has a total calorie budget. This budget can be divided into "essentials" and "extras."

With a financial budget, the essentials are items like rent and food. The extras are for things like cameras, movies, and vacations. In a calorie budget, the essentials are the minimum calories required to meet your nutrient needs. They are foods selected from the different food groups, such as milk, meat, beans, fruits, vegetables and grains.

Oils are not a food group, but you need some for good health.* The extras in your food budget are the calories you spend on alcohol and luxuries to make your food taste good. These luxuries are in solid fats, such as butter, chicken fat, beef fat, margarine, many cheeses, bacon, ice cream, and whole milk; added sugars, such as sugar, high fructose corn syrup, brown sugar, sucrose, syrups, honey, candy, cookies, and regular soft drinks. Extras may also be eating more foods from any food group than the food guide recommends. These are your discretionary calories.

The good news is that each person has an allowance for some discretionary calories based on estimated calorie needs by age/sex group and level of physical activity.

You can learn your portion size by customizing your own daily food plan at: http://www.choosemyplate.gov/myplate/index.aspx.

*The USDA Dietary Guidelines for Americans recommends that we get most of our fats from sources of polyunsaturated and monounsaturated fatty acids, such as fish, nuts, and vegetable oils.

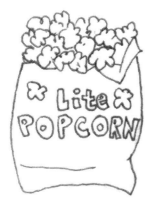

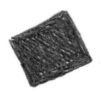

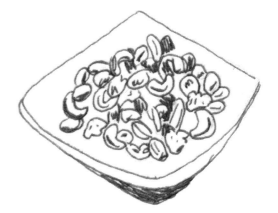

Why is physical activity important?

People of all ages can benefit from being physically active.

Being physically active can help you:
- Increase your chances of living longer
- Feel better about yourself
- Decrease your chances of becoming depressed
- Sleep well at night
- Move around more easily
- Have stronger muscles and bones
- Stay at, or get to, a healthy weight
- Be with friends or meet new people
- Enjoy yourself and have fun

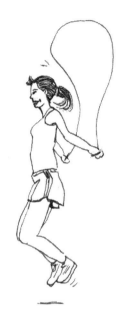

When you are not physically active, you are more likely to:
- Get heart disease
- Get type 2 diabetes
- Have high blood pressure
- Have high cholesterol
- Have a stroke

Some types of physical activity are especially beneficial:

- *Aerobic activities* make you breathe harder and makes your heart beat faster. Aerobic activities can be moderate or vigorous in their intensity.

- *Muscle-strengthening* activities make your muscles stronger. These include activities like push-ups and lifting weights. It is important to work all the different parts of the body—your legs, hips, back, chest, stomach, shoulders and arms.

- *Bone-strengthening activities* make your bones stronger. Bone strengthening activities, like jumping, are especially important for children and adolescents. These activities produce a force on the bones that promotes bone growth and strength.

- *Balance and stretching activities* enhance physical stability and flexibility, which reduces risk of injuries. Examples are gentle stretching, dancing, yoga, martial arts, and tai chi.

Adapted from: *USDA, Physical Activity:* "Why is Physical Activity Important?" November 9, 2012.

Good Ingredients Make You Want to Purr

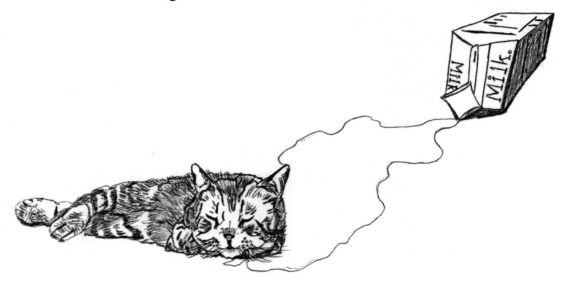

Buy organic milk. It is free of growth hormones, antibiotics, and dangerous pesticides. It also tastes better; even the fat free is delicious and creamy.

Vanilla soy milk makes fabulous shakes. My favorite brands are: Silk, made by White Wave; and Eden. There are also some generic brands that are good; just be sure they are fortified with vitamins and minerals, and made with non-genetically modified soybeans.

Medjool dates, originally from the Middle East, are available in bulk at most supermarkets. They are plump, soft and delicious. You only need one or two for great flavor. Try them for dessert in place of cookies or candy. Larger quantities can be stored in the freezer. Just remember to remove the pit.

Fresh figs are amazing in shakes. Sample the different varieties as they come into season late summer and fall. My favorites are the Black Mission, Gold Mecca, and Brown Turkey varieties.

"There are four types of pineapples mainly found in the marketplace. These include the Gold, smooth Cayenne, Red Spanish and Sugar Loaf. The Gold variety features an extra sweet flavor, golden color, and higher vitamin C content."

Buy nuts that are unsalted and have no other ingredients added.

Purchase only pure honey, and try to support your local bee keepers, if possible. The darker the honey, the more intense the flavor.

Save wintering songbirds that make their homes in Central and South America by buying shade grown coffee that is organic.

Shop smart. Buy quality fruit in season, taking advantage of specials.
Remember, there is no waste when you freeze.

A Sweet Tooth

If you have a sweet tooth like my grandson, you will probably like cream of coconut or honey in your shakes.

Honey is always stored on the shelf in a tight container. An occasional stirring will prevent it from crystallizing. Honey is especially nice with fruit that tends to be a little tart.

Cream of coconut is used in several of my shakes because it's unique and rich flavor pairs well with certain fruits. After opening the can, empty contents into a small tight container and store in the refrigerator. It will keep for several months.

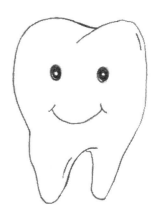

You can certainly interchange them to please your own taste, but keep in mind they are <u>discretionary</u> calories and should be used in moderation. One teaspoon should satisfy the most demanding sweet tooth.

CHAPTER 2

Tips and Techniques

Tips for Making Great Shakes

Easy Does It

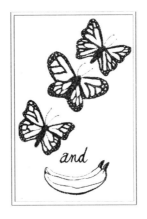

Tips for Making Great Shakes

Always ripen fruit at room temperature before refrigerating or freezing.

Pay attention to fruit while it is ripening. Handle with care.

Fruits are at their peak flavor and nutrition when fully ripened.

Bananas are ready when no green remains on the stem end and the peel is well mottled.

Mangos should be firm, but yield when gently pressed. Fragrance at the stem end, rather than color, is also an indication of how ripe and sweet the fruit may be. An exception to this is the recently popular variety of mango, the Ataulfo, that when fully ripe turns from green to golden yellow.

Select strawberries that are fragrant and bright red. They are store ready.

Pineapples are ripe when fragrant and the center leaves are easy to pull out. A good pineapple will be firm and plump with leaves that show no signs of dryness. Avoid any that have brown spots or bruises.

Peaches are ready when fragrant, and background color has no green remaining. "The amount of red blush on fruit depends on the variety, and is not always a sign of ripeness."

Blueberries, raspberries, blackberries and grapes are always store ready.

Figs are ripe when fruit is soft to the touch. Use or freeze immediately.

Some Nutty Advice

> Because of their high fat content, both shelled and unshelled nuts should be stored in the refrigerator or freezer if kept over a long period of time. This will prevent them from becoming rancid.

EASY DOES IT

Freezing Fruit for Fabulous Shakes

All fresh fruit should be thoroughly washed before peeling, except, of course, bananas.

Peel <u>only</u> bananas, pineapple and mangos. Remove stems from figs and grapes.

Gently rinse and drain berries, grapes and figs in cold water:
1) Spread fruit over paper-lined cookie sheet to dry.
2) With sharp knife, carefully remove green caps on strawberries.
3) Measure fruit in 4-ounce increments and place in <u>individual</u> snack, ziplock bags.

Larger fruit should be cut in small chunks:
1) Bananas are always in 3-ounce increment packages.
2) All other fruit should be in 4-ounce increments.
3) After measuring, place fruit in <u>individual</u> snack, ziplock bags.

Group all packages together into <u>one large community ziplock</u> for easy access. Freeze immediately.

Remove as much air as possible from the freezer bag before closing. "Most frozen fruits maintain high quality for 8 to12 months."

CHAPTER 3

The Shake Connection

Tools of the Trade

Make Friends with Your Blender

How Sweet it Is

Shop Smart Share the Prep

Tools for Making Great Shakes

Share a Shake

Adult supervision is necessary when any appliance is used by, or near, young children.

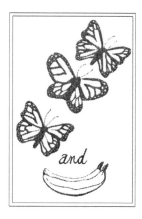

Tools of the Trade

Most kitchens are already equipped to make these shakes. Nothing fancy is needed here. Below, I have listed what it takes to make the job simple and fun:

Blender - It is not necessary to have the top of the line. A 40 oz. capacity jar enables you to double all of these shakes. Most blenders come equipped with a pulse button, highly recommended here for processing frozen fruit. It is important to read the enclosed instructions as you would with any other appliance.

small cutting board

kitchen scale

sharp paring knife

broad plastic spatula

serrated dinner knife

sturdy, long plastic tool*

measuring spoons

a happy spirit

* Melamine chopsticks—
available at most Chinese markets—also on-line.

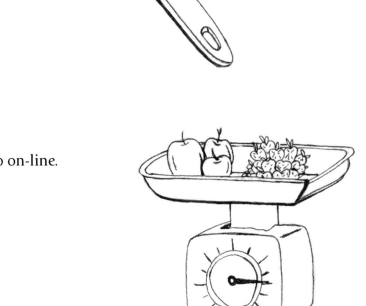

MAKE FRIENDS WITH YOUR BLENDER

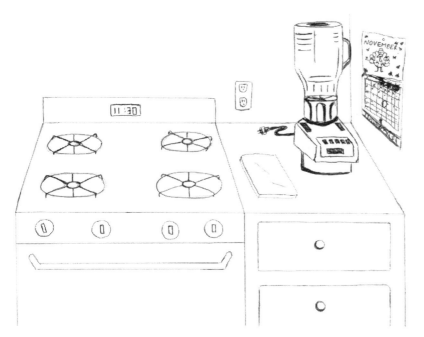

It is always a good idea to position any appliance you use often where it is handy and easy to get to. Consider placing your blender on the counter rather than inside a cabinet. You will then be sure to make these shakes often with ease and enjoyment.

After you have become friends with your blender, you will want to know which speed button is recommended for processing frozen fruit with liquid. This will ensure a speedy and smooth result every time. Refer to your blender's manual.

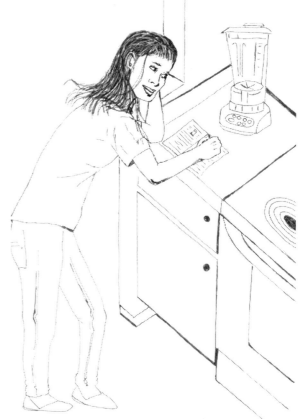

A Word of Caution:

Do not let the motor run if there is nothing moving. This can harm the motor. Turn off the blender, remove the lid, and stir with your sturdy plastic tool. Place lid back on the blender jar and continue processing.

HOW SWEET IT IS

Once you have stocked your kitchen with the key ingredients, you will always be able to **make a shake.** You will not have to make frequent trips to the grocery store--**a delicious and nourishing snack** will always be at your fingertips. That is because the entire premise for this book is one of simplicity and ease. Although there are 18 different shakes, most of the ingredients are already in your kitchen. By shopping smart you will be taking advantage of the specials on fruit as they come into season. But don't overlook the nuts and seeds--they are an excellent way to put variety into your diet.

Here is a list of the ingredients to make all of the shakes:

- fruit
- soy milk or milk*
- dates
- almonds
- sunflower seeds
- pistachios
- quick-rolled oats
- honey
- cream of coconut
- cocoa
- coffee
- walnuts
- Peanut Butter

How sweet it is!

*Children up to two years old should drink whole milk.

Allowing family members to help with chores is always a good way to lighten your load, while at the same time encourages teamwork, responsibility, and consideration of others.

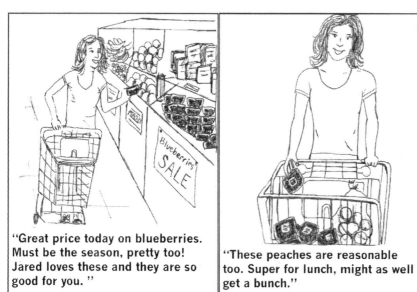

"Great price today on blueberries. Must be the season, pretty too! Jared loves these and they are so good for you."

"These peaches are reasonable too. Super for lunch, might as well get a bunch."

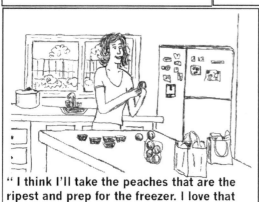

" I think I'll take the peaches that are the ripest and prep for the freezer. I love that Butterfly shake with the walnuts."

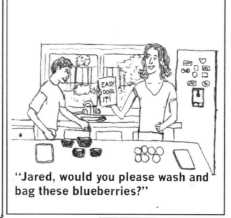

"Jared, would you please wash and bag these blueberries?"

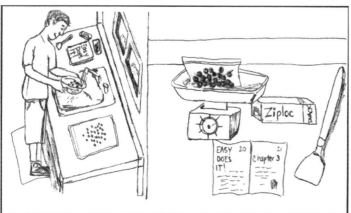

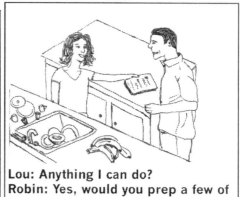

Lou: Anything I can do?
Robin: Yes, would you prep a few of those ripe bananas for our shakes?

Tools for Making Great Shakes:

Eyes to see with

Hands to work with

Ears to hear with

Mouth to taste with

Friends to share with

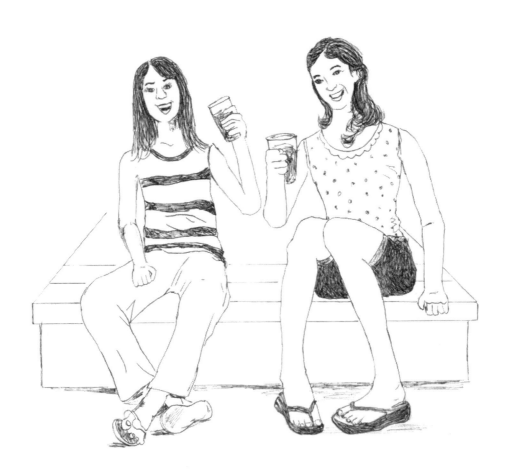

Share a Shake

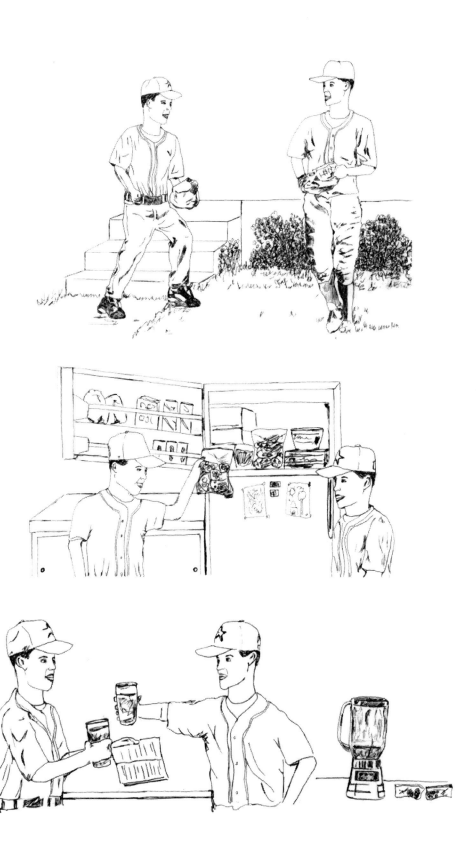

CHAPTER 4

Make a Shake

A Message to the Kids

Marilyn's Great Workout Shake

Index of Forest Shakes

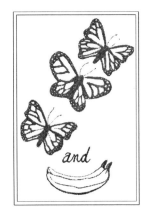

A Message to the Kids

When you make your shake, notice the pretty colors as they unfold and twirl in front of you. Know that the sun, rain, soil, trees, air and animals are inside your shake. Surround yourself with nature, simply to watch and listen to its sound.

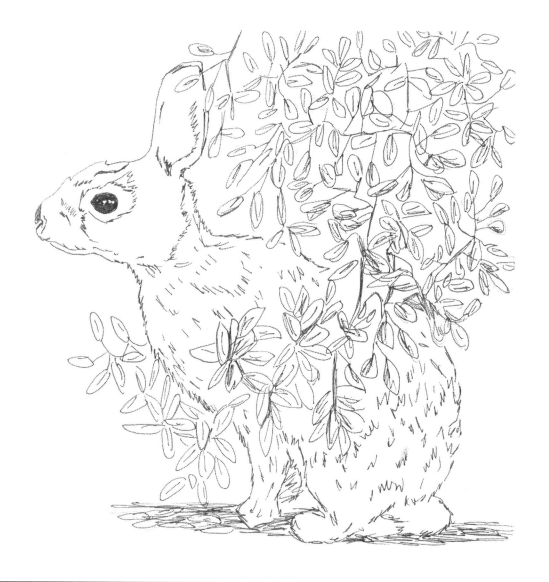

Marilyn's Great Workout Shake

3 ounces frozen banana - cut into ½-inch pieces
4 ounces frozen mango - cut into ½-inch pieces
1/3 cup of quick cooking rolled oats
1 cup vanilla soy milk or 1% milk
1 teaspoon cream of coconut

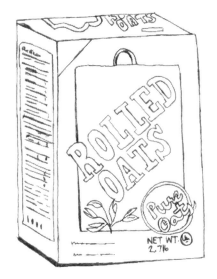

Pour liquid into blender jar.

Add oatmeal, fruit, and cream of coconut

Separate ingredients with a sturdy plastic tool.

Return lid to blender jar. <u>Pulse</u> in short bursts about 10 times.

Turn off pulse button and process until smooth, about 20 seconds.

What a way to start the day. If you like **oatmeal** you will love this shake: thick, creamy and delicious! With this nutritional powerhouse you're bound for a great ride, whether walking, swimming or biking—just like the champion racehorse, Seabiscuit—out front and winning.

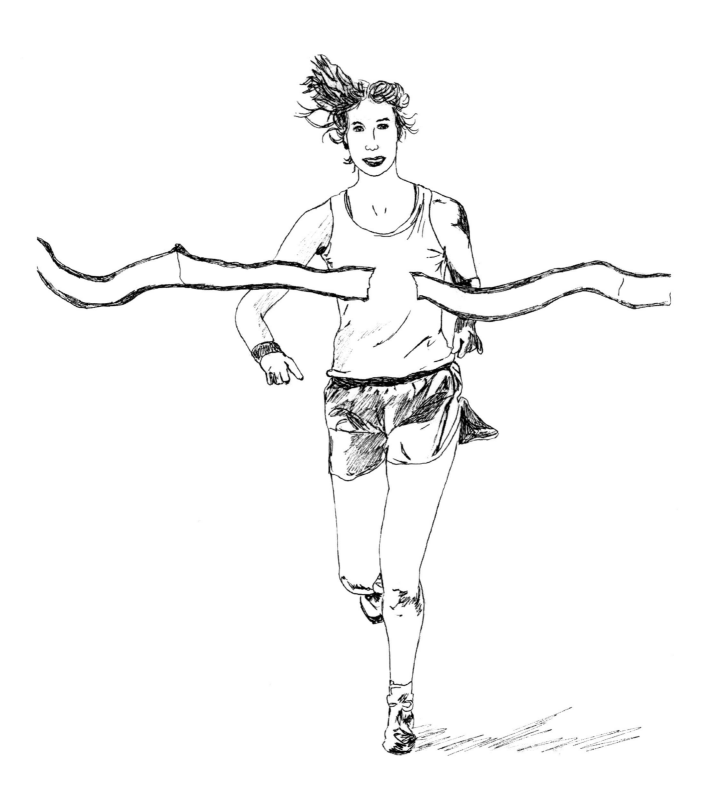

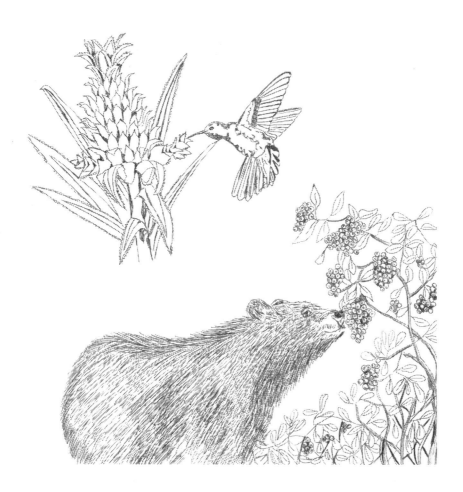

We are not the only ones enjoying nature's bounty. While we are feasting on the fruits of the season, many of our wildlife are devouring it, too.

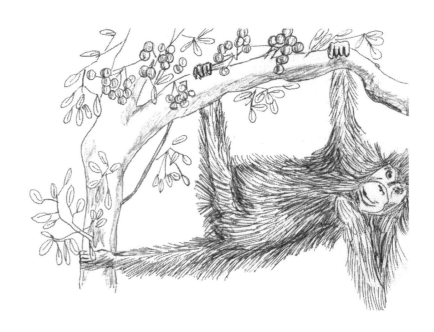

These shakes are not recommended for children under one.

All shakes include bananas.

FOREST SHAKES

26   Black Bear................ blueberries
28   Bat ....mango
30   Bee ....strawberries
32   Hummingbird..........pineapple
34   Orangutan.....................figs
36   Cardinal ....raspberries & dates
38   Chickadee............sunflower seeds & grapes
40   Antelope......chocolate and raspberries
42   Butterfly.............. peaches and walnuts
44   Raccoon.......................grapes
46   Peacock.................blackberries
48   Monkey Latte....... coffee and dates

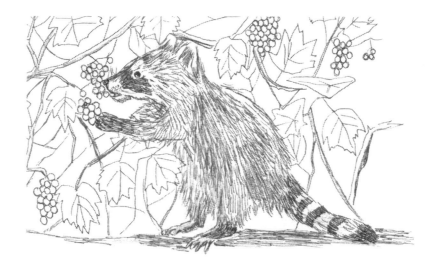

"When one tugs at a single thing in nature, he finds it attached to the rest of the world."—- John Muir.

FOREST DESSERT SHAKES

50   Parrot....................pistachio date
52   Chipmunk.............. chocolate almond
54   Monkey...................banana date.
56   Squirrel................chocolate peanut butter
58   Spunky Monkey........chocolate coffee

The Black Bear

3 ounces frozen banana - cut into ½-inch
pieces
4 ounces frozen blueberries
8 ounces vanilla soy milk or 1% milk
1 teaspoon honey

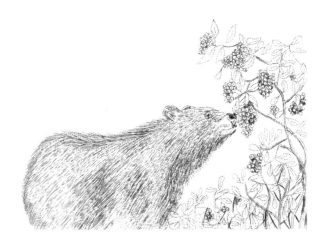

Measure liquid into blender jar. Add fruit and
honey. Separate fruit with a sturdy plastic tool.
Return lid to blender jar. Pulse in short bursts
about 8 to10 times. Turn off pulse button and
process until smooth, a matter of seconds.

Wild blueberries have been around for hundreds of years in North America, and were enjoyed
by early explorers for their rich and unique flavor. Lewis and Clarke dined on blueberries and
venison with the Indians during their famous expedition through the Northwest. They were
smart to eat them, because blueberries are an exciting nutritional story. The secret lies in its
deep, purple-blue color, produced by anthocyanins––antioxidants—which leading health
authorities claim may reduce the risk of certain diseases and combat some of the effects of
aging. You may not get to share your blueberries with the Native Americans, but you certainly
can enjoy them with your family and friends. While shopping, always look for plump firm
berries with a silver sheen. Remember, they only last a few days in the refrigerator, so buy plenty for the freezer to enjoy year round.

First Class Hibernator

The American black bear is the smallest North American bear. Though classified as a carnivore, it is in actuality an omnivore, whose diet varies throughout the year. Its main food source comes mostly from plants, but it also eats medium-sized mammals, fish and insects. In the fall, black bear can be found gorging on fruits, nuts and acorns, which gives them sufficient reserves to prepare for hibernation in the winter when less food is available to them.

Black bear often raid honey combs, adding even more carbohydrates to their diet, but it is really the bees and larvae they are after. The honey is dessert.

"Female bear give birth during hibernation and nurse their cubs through a period of helplessness." She will not leave the den, unless disturbed, and emerges in the spring strong and healthy. "By that time the cubs can walk and follow the mother as she feeds."

Animals like the bear **transport seeds** in their fur and droppings. This is one of the ways plants ensure they will continue to live on earth.

Black bear also play an ecological role as **scavengers**, consuming carrion, which is then recycled into nutrients.

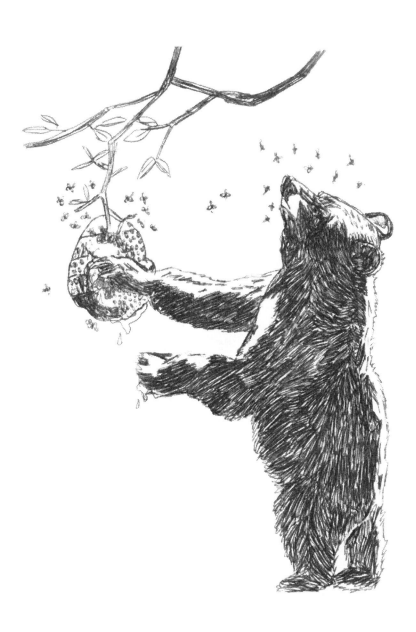

The Bat

3 ounces frozen banana - cut into ½-inch pieces
4 ounces frozen mango - cut into ½-inch pieces
8 ounces vanilla soy milk or 1% milk
1 teaspoon cream of coconut

Measure liquid into blender. Add fruit and cream of coconut. Separate fruit with a sturdy plastic tool. Return lid to blender jar. Pulse in short bursts about 8 to10 times. Turn off pulse button and process until smooth, a matter of seconds.

Though it may come as a surprise to learn: More **mangos** are eaten fresh around the world than any other fruit; more than the banana and the apple.

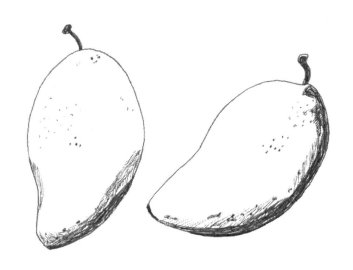

Mangos were first cultivated in India about 4,000 years ago where they were brought to other tropical countries by European explorers. Today, they are grown throughout the world in most tropical regions, often serving as the main food source.

Mangos are an excellent source of antioxidants. A serving size (1/2 cup), with only 50 calories, gives you 15% of your daily value requirements for vitamin A, plus a whopping 40% for vitamin C.

Because of their sweet and rich flavor, mangos are often used in exotic salsas, salads and desserts.* For a simple hearty breakfast toss them on your cereal, and be sure to keep plenty in the freezer so you can enjoy them all year round.

*In the 6th chapter of *Recipes for Vibrant Living*, check out two luscious recipes where I have used mango as a salad and a main course.

Nature's No. 1 Pest Controller

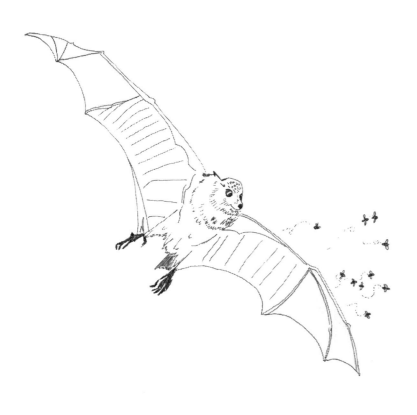

Probably no animal on this planet is as misunderstood, yet so vital to the ecosystem, as the bat.

Bats do not get tangled in the hair, nor are they blind or vicious. "Bats very rarely carry rabies. In fact, more than 99% in the wild do not carry the disease. Bats fly high, so if you see one on the ground it may have a broken wing or could be sick with a disease. You do not want to touch it."

There are no vampire bats in North America; they are in southern Mexico, Central and South America, where they feed on host animals. Most of the bats in North America are insectivores. "A single little brown bat can eat more than 1,000 mosquito-sized insects in just one hour."

Did you know that a lot of our favorite fruits, such as bananas, avocados, dates, figs, peaches and mangos owe their existence to bat pollination; that fruit-eating bats are so effective at dispersing seed in the tropical forests they have been called "farmers of the tropics?"

And next time you are out enjoying a Margarita or Blue Agave Nectar on your French toast, thank the lesser long-nosed bat for pollinating and dispersing seeds of the Agave plant in Mexico.

Instead of disliking bats, let us celebrate them for the very important role they play in the environment.

Up-to-date and comprehensive information on bat education and conservation, can be obtained at: Bat Conservation International, P.O. Box 162603, Austin, TX 78716. (512) 327-9721 www.batcon.org/.

The Bee

3 ounces frozen banana - cut into ½-inch pieces
4 ounces of frozen strawberries - cut into ½-inch pieces
8 ounces vanilla soy milk or 1% milk
1 teaspoon honey

Measure liquid into blender jar.
Add fruit and honey. Separate
fruit with a sturdy plastic tool.
Return lid to blender jar. Pulse in
short bursts about 8 to 10 times.
Turn off pulse button and process
until smooth, a matter of seconds.

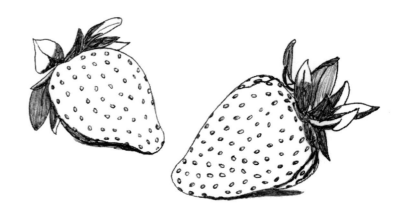

Strawberries rank high on the list
of favorite fruits of both adults
and children, giving this creamy
and delicious shake a big thumbs
up every time.

Strawberries, like most brightly colored berries, are exceptionally good for you. You may be
surprised to learn that just eight medium-size berries contain more vitamin C than an
orange—plus plenty of folic acid, fiber and potassium—all vital to the health and maintenance
of your body.

Strawberries actually taste best at room temperature, but in order to keep them longer they
should be stored dry in the refrigerator. Wash them just before serving, with their green caps on
and under a gentle spray of cool water. Allow them to drain; then place on paper towels to dry.
You can freeze the ones you don't eat right away by following instructions on the "Easy Does
It" page of this book.

Fruit trivia: Strawberries are the only fruit with seeds on the outside. "On average there are 200
seeds in a strawberry."

The Pollinator

Did you ever wonder how that plump round apple came to be on that tree? Marvel at those bright red strawberries sitting on your cereal? And what about those crunchy little almonds you just love to snack on?

Most of the food we eat is actually the work of a little organism even busier than we are. Why, and how does this happen? Let's begin with the flower.

The purpose of a flower is to reproduce. But it can't usually do it alone; it must have help. Enter the bee, a natural biological pollinator.

The bee needs something the flower can offer--nourishment. But the flower has to attract the bee first. In order to do this, it must:

- **Advertise**--by way of color, scent, and nectar guides. Many flowers also have UV patterns that attract bees, but are invisible to humans.

- **Provide a landing pad**--bees cannot hover in space like the hummingbird, another important pollinator.

- **Offer a reward**--food in the form of pollen and nectar.

Other important thing: Male bees are often attracted to flowers that look like a potential mate.

Now, this is where it gets sexy, or should I say sticky? The flower must show that it can provide a way for the pollen to be transferred to the bee, then to the stigma of another plant; fertilization can then take place and genetic information be exchanged. The result: a seed is produced and a new generation of plants appear.

Beelieve: Only honeybees make honey and beeswax. Honeybees must tap two million flowers to make one pound of honey.

There are no native North American honeybees. They were brought over by the early European settlers who needed beeswax as a means for producing candles and honey to sweeten their food.

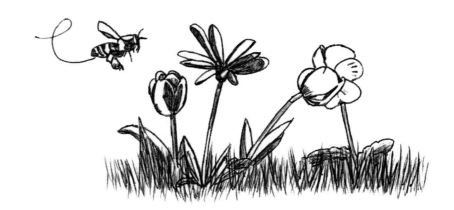

The Hummingbird

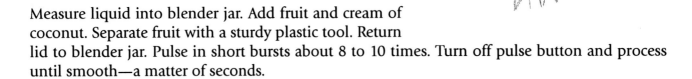

3 ounces frozen banana - cut into ½-inch pieces
4 ounces frozen pineapple - cut into ½-inch pieces
8 ounces vanilla soy milk or 1% milk
1 teaspoon cream of coconut

Measure liquid into blender jar. Add fruit and cream of
coconut. Separate fruit with a sturdy plastic tool. Return
lid to blender jar. Pulse in short bursts about 8 to 10 times. Turn off pulse button and process
until smooth—a matter of seconds.

Did you know? When you purchase a **pineapple** at the grocery store you are not only buying a
delicious and nourishing fruit, but also a very old symbol of international hospitality? This
story begins with Christopher Columbus and his arrival in the West Indies, discovering the
exotic looking fruit. They soon learned that the fruit is not only succulent and delicious, but
also a sign of welcome and friendship. When the explorers returned home, they brought the
fruit and its symbolism with them; it soon became an item of great popularity for centuries.

In Colonial America where sweets were quite rare and refrigeration on ships non-existent,
pineapples "that made the trip home and could still be eaten were very prized." To be given a
pineapple "was truly an honor;" likewise, a fresh pineapple displayed on the center of a dining
room table was considered a gesture of great cordiality.

There are other reasons for placing the pineapple on a pedestal: The sweet nature of the fruit
and the fact that it contains the enzyme "bromelain," credited for breaking down protein,
make it a very fine choice for a satisfying and healthy dessert. And it is an excellent source of
vitamin C.

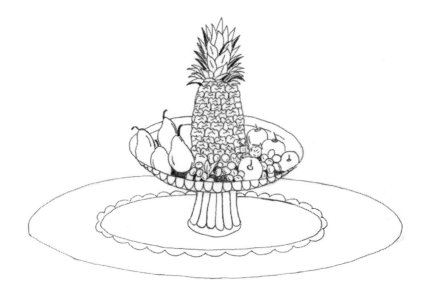

The Little Helicopter

Hummingbirds are very important pollinators of wildflowers in the continental United States. If they live in your area, you can attract them to your yard by planting colorful tubular-shaped flowers. The long slender bills on these tiny birds are especially designed to extract nectar from even the deepest throated flower.

Native plants require a lot less care compared to non-native plants, and the birds more often than not have co-evolved with them. What's more, native plants thrive without having to rely on pesticides and other potentially dangerous chemicals.

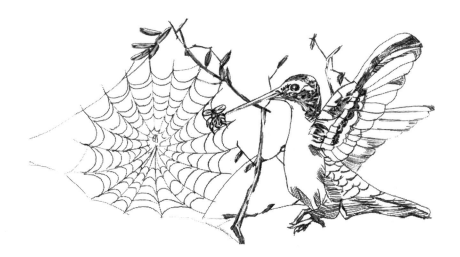

When planning your garden, you will want to consider both annual and perennials with different blooming periods. For migrating hummingbirds, find out what time of the year these birds usually arrive in your neighborhood and plant accordingly. Most nature centers and nurseries are very helpful sources for obtaining this kind of information.

But remember, all wildlife must have water. A bird bath with a few small rocks placed in it gives these little birds a chance to bathe---something they love to do—and provides a constant source of water for them. "Place the water container about 10 feet from dense shrubs or other cover that predators may use."

Hummingbirds supplement their diet with small insects, adding fat and protein to their carbohydrate diet; they are very adept at finding insects deep inside the flowers. They also seize insects from spider webs while hovering in space.

The Orangutan

3 ounces frozen banana - cut into ½-inch pieces
4 ounces frozen figs - cut into ½-inch pieces
8 ounces vanilla soy milk or 1% milk
1 teaspoon cream of coconut

Measure liquid into blender jar. Add fruit and coconut cream. Separate fruit with a sturdy plastic tool. Return lid to blender jar. Pulse in short bursts about 8 to 10 times. Turn off pulse button and process until smooth, a matter of seconds.

A native of the Mediterranean region, "the **fig** is one of the earliest fruits known to man," and the first fruit to be mentioned in the Bible. "It is estimated that they have been around for at least 6,000 years." Most of the figs you see today come from California, unless you just happen to have some growing in the yard, which in most cases are devoured by the birds before you ever have a chance to taste one.

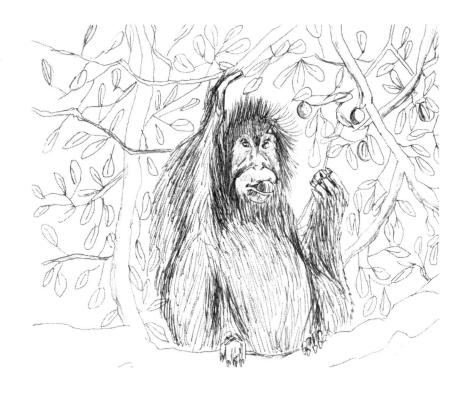

The season for figs is usually June through October, with the different varieties available at different times. An important thing to know about figs is that they should be eaten at their peak of ripeness when the fruit is plump and soft, allowing the sugar content and unique satiny texture to develop to its fullest. Also worth knowing: figs are an excellent source of potassium---important for helping to control blood pressure and keeping our muscles strong.

But you should also eat figs just for the taste. Prepare ahead of time and surprise your guests with this fabulous fig concoction. Spread the diced fruit in a single layer on a cookie sheet to harden in the freezer. When firm, place in ziplock bags to be used whenever you are ready.

Man of the Forest

How would you like to swing through the trees with an extra pair of hands, create your own tools, eat lots of fruit, and never have to come down to earth? If all this sounds appealing, you would probably enjoy being an orangutan.

Orangutans are large, red-haired apes that live in the tropical rainforests on the islands of Sumatra and Borneo. They are "highly intelligent" animals that can solve problems, grasp things with both hands and feet, craft their own tools, and turn leaves into umbrellas and cups for catching water. Their habitat is rich in biodiversity, and they know where to find their favorite fruit--fig or durian.

But all is not paradise in the rainforest. Orangutans are "critically endangered." Their predator is man. Although they "share 96.4% of our DNA," that 3.6% difference has pushed them off of the planet and onto the verge of extinction.

Although Indonesia's forests have been ranked as one of the richest in the world in species of both plants and animals, nature cannot compete with the pace of habitat destruction occurring in these hot spots. "Orangutans are gardeners of the forest. They play a crucial role in forest regeneration through the fruits and seeds they eat." As the forest goes, so go the birds, the reptiles, the amphibians, and the orangutan.

Leaders of three nations that share Borneo signed a declaration to save and maintain an 85,000 square mile area called the "Heart of Borneo," one of only two places in the world where rhinos, elephants, and orangutans coexist.

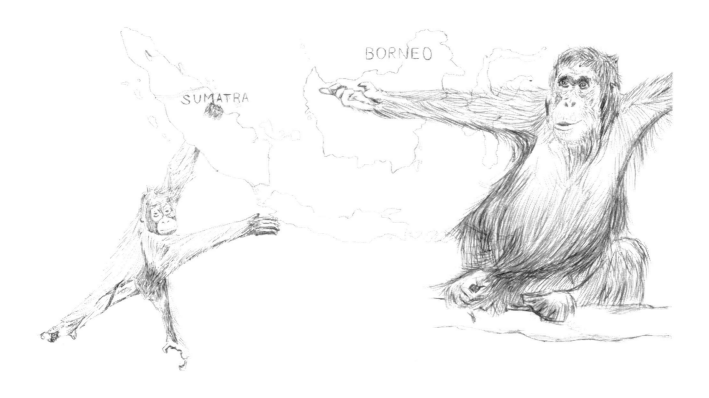

The Cardinal

3 ounces frozen banana - cut into ½-inch pieces
4 ounces frozen raspberries - allow a few minutes to separate
1 or 2 dates (seeds removed) diced in ¼-inch pieces
8 ounces vanilla soy milk or 1% milk

Measure liquid into blender
jar. Add fruit. Separate fruit
with a sturdy plastic tool.
Return lid to blender jar.
Pulse in short bursts about 8
to 10 times. Turn off pulse
button and process until
smooth, a matter of seconds.

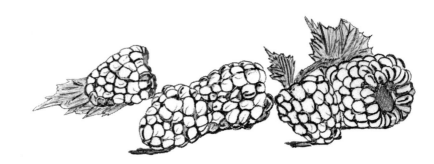

Tangy, tart and delicious, the **raspberry** is the most delicate of all the berries. The reason for
that lies in the center of the fruit, which is hollow. Since they are so perishable, raspberries
should be kept dry while in the refrigerator, and eaten within a few days. Wash them only
before using or freezing, following directions on the "Easy Does It" page of your book.

Like all deep-colored berries, raspberries are an excellent source of vitamin C with just 1/2 cup
providing 50% of our daily value requirement. They are also an excellent source of fiber.

Raspberries are expensive. When shopping in the grocery stores, take advantage of seasonal
sales. Look for berries that are medium to bright red and in unstained cartons; they will taste
better and hold up longer.

The Performer

The Northern Cardinal, with its brilliant red plumage and cheerful disposition, is probably the most loved songbird in North America. So popular is the cardinal that seven states have adopted it as their state bird.

Cardinals have many admirable traits:

They are monogamous (meaning they have one mate) and remain together throughout the year.

As the breeding season approaches in the spring, the male turns his attention to his mate. He will offer her a seed, and beak to beak she accepts his gift. This enchanting act is known as the "cardinal kiss."

Cardinals are altricial (hatched with eyes closed and completely dependent on their parents). Both parents feed the chicks a diet of insects from the moment they hatch, and continue for a period of "25 to 56 days after they fledge from the nest."

Northern Cardinals love to sing; even the female sings—one of the few female North American songbirds that does. Since they do not migrate (and happen to live in your area), why not attract them to your yard by providing a habitat for them? You can then be a witness to their tender rituals and enjoy their beautiful song all year long. Just remember the four things all wildlife need to survive: food, water, shelter and space.

Cardinals "are valued as destroyers of weed seeds."

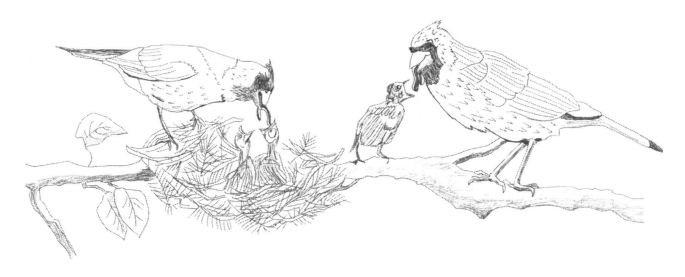

The Chickadee

3 ounces frozen banana - cut into ½-inch pieces
4 ounces frozen seedless green grapes - cut into ½-inch pieces
2 rounded Tablespoons sunflower seeds
8 ounces vanilla soy milk or 1% milk
1 teaspoon cream of coconut

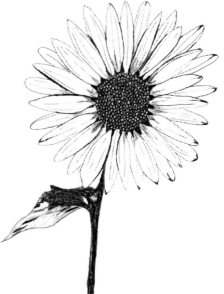

Place sunflower seeds in blender jar.
Return lid and process until finely ground.
Turn off blender. Place liquid, fruit, and cream of
coconut in blender jar. Separate fruit with a sturdy
plastic tool. Return lid and pulse about 8 to 10 times.
Turn off pulse button and process until smooth, a matter of seconds.

.

Sunflower seeds come from the center of a tall and
showy flower native to North America. Many of us are
familiar with the famous painting of sunflowers by the
Dutch artist, Vincent Van Gogh.

Sunflower seeds are a powerhouse of nutrition--"1/4
cup provides 90.5% of your daily value requirement for
vitamin E," just one of the essential nutrients your body requires to stay healthy and can't
manufacturer on its own, depending on plants to obtain it.

Sunflower seeds are also rich in protein, minerals, and healthy fats, making them a great source
of energy, which is why the birds flock to them.

The Acrobat

Chickadees can be found in the forest canopies gleefully foraging for insects. They often hang upside down while feeding on their prey. They are highly energetic birds, with huge appetites, known for putting a sizable dent in the insect population.

These acrobatic little birds also like sunflower seeds. If they live in your neighborhood, you can attract them to your yard with a bird feeder, where they will patiently take their turn.

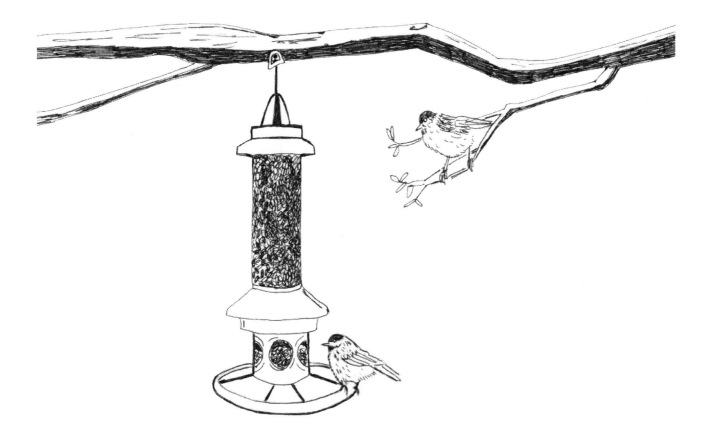

Chickadees favor the black oil variety of sunflower seed, readily available at many nurseries, nature centers, and supermarkets. It is best to purchase seed at places that have a fast turnover. Seed stored for long periods of time can become rancid.

Chickadees have one of the most sophisticated and varied call systems of any feeder bird--a reason to entice them. Just remember to keep the feeder clean.

The Antelope

3 ounces frozen banana - cut into ½-inch pieces
4 ounces frozen red raspberries - allow a few minutes to separate
8 ounces chocolate soy milk or 1% milk + 2 Tablespoons cocoa
1 teaspoon honey - optional

Measure liquid into blender jar. Add fruit and cocoa (if using). Separate fruit with a sturdy plastic tool. Return lid to blender jar. Pulse in short bursts about 8 to 10 times. Turn off pulse button and process until smooth, a matter of seconds.

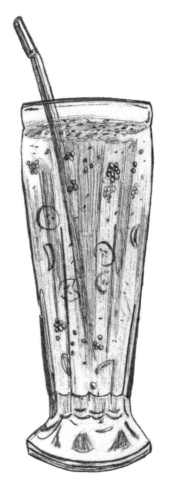

Because of their rich content of vitamin C, potassium and fiber, **raspberries** were important as a late summer food source for the Native Americans, early pioneers, and wildlife. Today, they are used creatively by gourmet dessert chefs, often combining them with chocolate. You don't have to go very far to get the same results. Here they are paired with **chocolate** and **banana** to make this simple but delicious shake. It's like eating a healthy banana split with a straw.

The reason raspberries are hollow in the center is because at harvest the central core of the berry remains on the bush. This is in contrast to the plump blackberry that gives up the core along with the berry.

The Athlete

The Greater Kudu, one of the most beautiful and spectacular animals of the antelope family, has the amazing ability to jump as high, and sometimes even higher, than eight feet. This capability is one of its "best defense strategies" against predators. Like an Olympic high jumper, it escapes the cheetah, lion, leopard, and other serious enemies by leaping over tall bushes.

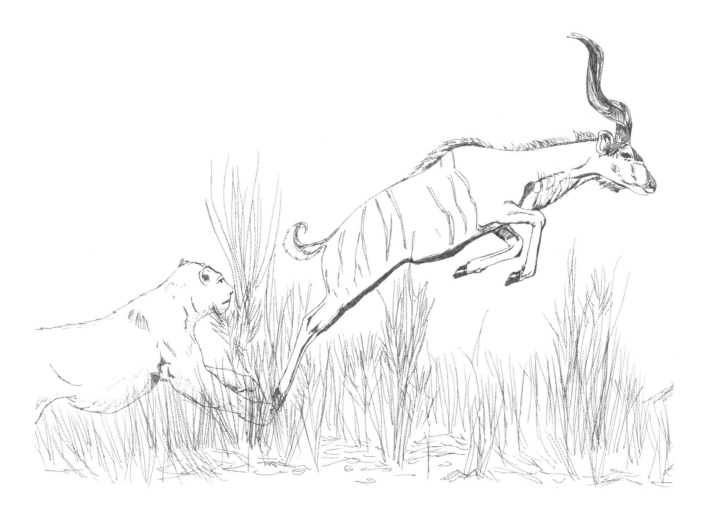

These herbivores are able to live in the dryer parts of eastern and southern Africa, owing to certain physical adaptations—evolved traits which make them capable of going several days without drinking water. They also draw in liquid from the plants and fruits they eat, such as watermelon and berries.

Unlike deer that shed its antlers, kudus keep their horns for life. Only the bull (male) grows graceful, spiraling horns, which can sometimes reach a height of six feet.

The Butterfly

3 ounces frozen banana - cut into ½-inch pieces
4 ounces frozen peaches - cut into ½-inch pieces
2 rounded Tablespoons walnut pieces
8 ounces vanilla soy milk or 1% milk
1 teaspoon honey

Place walnuts in blender jar. Return lid and process until finely ground. Turn off blender. Place liquid, fruit and honey in blender jar. Separate fruit with a sturdy plastic tool. Return lid and pulse about 8 to 10 times. Turn off pulse button and process until smooth, a matter of seconds.

When I return from my workout at the gym, I am ready for a delicious and refreshing little meal. I also want something extra nourishing to replenish and repair my body, like "The Butterfly" shake. This synergistic combination keeps my body humming! When summer rolls around, I am ready to do some serious peach shopping. I like to buy peaches when they are still a little firm and slightly fragrant. That way I can place them in a bowl on my table to be eaten as they ripen. Peaches ripen and taste best at room temperature.

Peaches are not only a good source of antioxidants A and C, but also low in calories--a great reason to take advantage of seasonal sales; remember, by freezing there is no waste here, and you get to enjoy this incredible shake all year.

The Transformer

If you have a sunny spot in your yard, why not create a butterfly garden? It is a very therapeutic and rewarding way to spend some time outdoors—you will also be helping the environment. "Butterflies suffer from the same ills that plague all wildlife these days: habitat loss, pollution, invasive species, and global warming."

To attract wildlife the first thing to consider are their immediate basic needs: food, water, shelter and space. When considering food, choose native species—"generations of butterflies have taste-tested them—"and you're more likely to have better results. The plants will be happier, too. Also keep in mind: adults (butterflies) eat nectar and larvae (caterpillars) eat plants. Sometimes the same plant will provide food for both, but not always. "Most butterfly caterpillars are very persnickety eaters; some eat only one kind of plant." A well-known example of this is the Monarch butterfly, who always deposit her eggs on the milkweed plant, the only plant her offspring will eat.

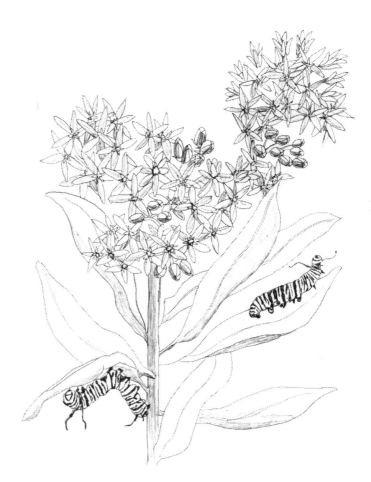

When beginning any new project, it is always wise to do a little homework first. Your local library, nature center, and native plant society are all excellent sources for obtaining all of the information you will need.

Create a haven for butterflies—be witness to what is probably the most astonishing act in all of nature: the metamorphosis of the butterfly.

Did you know that with just a few qualifications you can have your garden certified by the National Wildlife Federation as a sanctuary for native wildlife in your area? Find out how at: http://www.nwf.org/How-to-Help/Garden-for-Wildlife/Create-a-Habitat.aspx.

The Raccoon

3 ounces frozen banana - cut into ½-inch pieces
4 ounces frozen seedless red or black grapes
8 ounces vanilla soy milk or 1% milk
1 teaspoon honey

Measure liquid into blender jar. Add fruit and honey. Separate fruit with a sturdy plastic tool. Return lid to blender jar. Pulse in short bursts about 8 to10 times. Turn off pulse button and process until smooth, a matter of seconds.

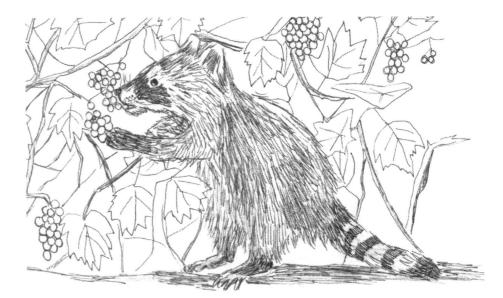

Were you aware that **grapes** are true berries? Did you know that grapes are one of the first fruits to be mentioned in the Bible?

What's in it for you? "Berries are some of the most nutritious fruits available. In addition to having a lot of vitamin C, folic acid, and dietary fiber, they have other plant chemicals that are very important to our health."

"The pigment that gives the dark blue, red, and purple colors to some berries, slows down or prevents damage to the body's cells."

So here are a few creative ways that you can eat grapes:

- Pair grapes with walnuts or pecans in chicken or tuna salad.

- Add grapes to spinach salads and toss with your favorite vinaigrette.

- Eat grapes frozen--tastes like a popsicle. Children absolutely love them this way.

For directions on preparing berries for the freezer, visit page 12.

On Behalf of the Raccoon

You most likely have come in contact with a raccoon. Its natural habitat is broad and diverse, ranging from marshes, ponds, mudflats, forests and riparian areas. They make their homes above the ground in hollowed-out tree cavities and abandoned ground burrows. Although raccoons are basically nocturnal animals, they will sometimes appear during the day if hungry.

Since we have encroached on their natural environment, many raccoons have taken up residency in urban neighborhoods. Although this little masked bandit can cause plenty of mischief, we need to respect its ecological niche as a predator to many rodents, other small animals, and distributor of seed.

So here are some questions we need to ask:

Do raccoons need handouts? Definitely not. The raccoon's natural diet is also diverse. They are omnivores, who are very clever opportunistic animals "capable of traveling great distances to find food" that is part of their natural diet. "They eat insects, nuts, worms, frogs, shellfish, fish, mammals, birds, eggs, grubs, snakes and fruit." They should be allowed to live their own wild lives and hunt for their own food, which is much better for them. Always remember, when you habituate wild animals to become dependent on you, those animals are no longer wild.

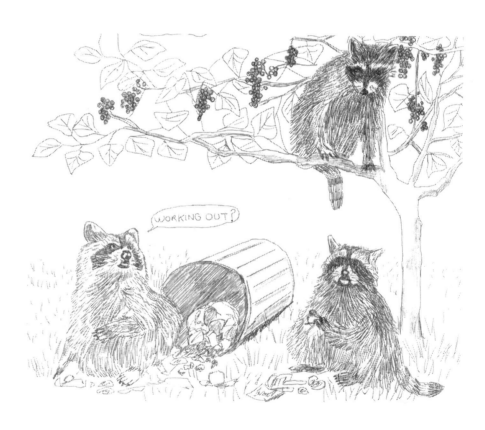

What should I do if a raccoon is raiding my garbage can?
"Garbage cans should be secured tightly to prevent a raccoon's access. You can fasten the lid securely with rope, bungee cords or weights. Garbage cans can be secured to a wooden stake or wall to prevent being knocked over. Commercial repellants can also be sprayed directly onto garbage cans to deter raccoons."

If you need suggestions or help with other problems concerning raccoons, you can call your city's Department of Fish and Wildlife.

The Peacock

3 ounces frozen banana - cut into ½-inch pieces
4 ounces frozen blackberries - allow to separate a little
8 ounces vanilla soy milk or 1% milk
1 teaspoon honey

Measure liquid into blender jar. Add fruit and honey. Separate fruit with a sturdy plastic tool. Return lid to blender jar. Pulse in short bursts about 8 to 10 times. Turn off pulse button and process until smooth, a matter of seconds.

Berries taste best in season—usually the warmer months of the year. Whether you buy them from the local growers, the stores, or are lucky enough to harvest yourself, seasonal berries offer more flavor and value.

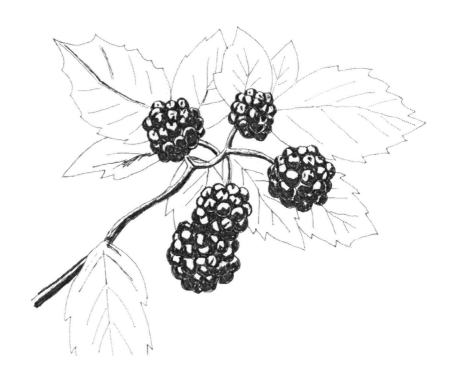

Blackberries are often overlooked because of their tiny seeds. It is these seeds that are a rich source of soluble fiber, responsible for supporting healthy blood sugar levels, and helping to keep our cholesterol and triglyceride levels in the normal range. The deep purple color in these berries points to anthocyanins--antioxidants which many scientists believe offer significant disease fighting protection.

So don't pass up these shiny plump berries when they appear in season. Remember, most blackberries have a shelf life of just a few days. Freezing should be done immediately to retain most of their fresh fruit quality. For tips on freezing berries, check out the "East Does It" page.

The beautiful blue peacock is the national bird of India and Sri Lanka. Only the male has the incredible tail and owns the name of peacock.

The female bird is called a peahen, and the young are called peachicks. Together they are known as peafowls. The natural habitat of the peafowl is the "dry semi-desert grassland, scrub, and deciduous forest. It forages and nests on the ground, but roosts on top of trees."

Don't mess with me! When encountering a serious predator, these birds will emit a "screaming alarm cry" to warn other animals that an enemy is approaching.

It knows when to strut and when to flee. At a minute's notice, they will take to the trees in "strong short bursts," sometimes with their chicks on their backs.

They eat from all the food groups. In the wild they "will eat nearly anything, but mainly feed on fruit, insects, worms, and occasionally snakes and mice."

The peacock is a good guy at heart! In domestic communities they are revered for their valuable role in the food web as a predator to young cobras.

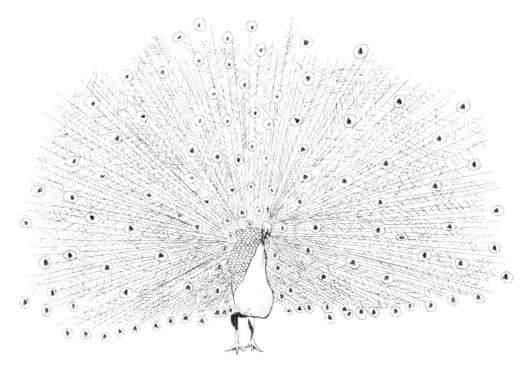

Who will make the cut? "Females are said to choose their mates according to the size, color, and quality of their outrageous feather trains." This is in keeping with the famous naturalist Charles Darwin's theory that all birds engage in sexual selection. "Darwin was right all along. In all sorts of species, from fish and birds to insects and frogs, females approach the males with the most elaborate displays and invite them to mate."

This shake is not recommended for young children.

Monkey Latte

6ounces frozen banana - cut into ½-inch pieces
8 ounces vanilla soy milk or 1% milk
2 Tablespoons espresso coffee beans
1 to 2 dates (seeds removed) diced in ¼-inch pieces

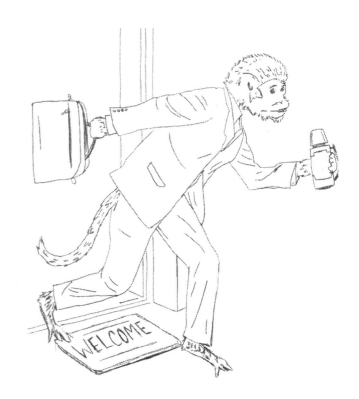

Measure liquid into blender jar. Add the rest of ingredients. Separate fruit with a sturdy plastic tool. Return lid to blender jar. Pulse in short bursts about 10 to 12 times. Turn off pulse button and process until smooth, a matter of seconds.

This is the ultimate wake-up-breakfast to go. Just pour it into a thermos and you're out the door.

The minuscule **coffee** chips burst with flavor in this yummy combination of bananas and dates, and it takes only a few minutes to prepare. Clean up time is equally fast. Just:

1. Fill empty jar 2/3 with water.
2. Add a few drops of detergent.
3. Give it a whirl.
4. Unplug, rinse with clear water.
5. Done!

Great news: It's now being touted by those in the know, that **coffee** "provides more healthful antioxidants than any other food or beverage in the American diet." But don't get carried away! Caffeine can make you jittery. It is also addictive. If you are one that needs a little nudge in the morning but are sensitive to caffeine, try this: mix up a batch of ground coffee made with half regular and half decaf.

More goodness here: bananas and dates are both excellent sources of soluble fiber, considered helpful in maintaining good blood sugar levels. Who wouldn't want that?

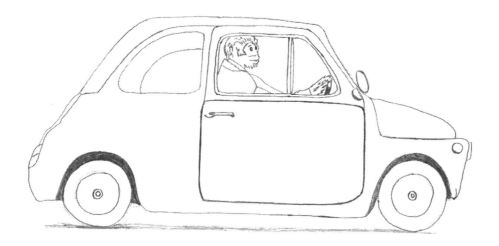

The Parrot

6 ounces frozen bananas - cut into ½-inch pieces
2 Tablespoons unsalted pistachios
1 or 2 dates (seeds removed) diced in ¼-inch pieces
8 ounces vanilla soy milk or 1% milk

Place pistachios in blender jar. Return lid and process until finely ground. Turn off blender. Place liquid, bananas and dates in blender jar. Separate fruit with a sturdy plastic tool. Return lid and pulse in short bursts about 8 to10 times.

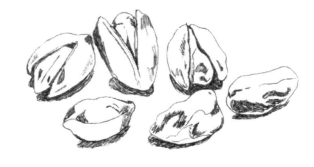

Turn off pulse button and process until smooth, a matter of seconds.

Nuts are a great way to add protein and other important nutrients to our diet without cholesterol and high levels of unhealthy fats. Equally as important, nuts seem to satisfy our craving for something rich and delicious. That is why I'm nuts about nuts!

Pistachios are not really nuts, but seeds of the cashew family, which includes sumac, mangos, and (no kidding here) poison ivy. They are native to Iran, the largest producer of pistachios in the world. "The second largest producer on the planet" is California.

Dates add sweetness and lots of exotic flavor to desserts. They are Mother Nature's treat to us in the form of complex carbohydrates. Complex carbohydrates are our body's best energy source. Dates are also an excellent source of fiber and potassium, both beneficial to our bodies in very different ways.

There are plenty of calories in this shake, but we all deserve a treat now and then; it's what helps us stay on track. Mindful eating is not about depriving ourselves; it is about awareness that "input" should not exceed "output." It is experiencing and enjoying "real" food.

The Mimic

What you should know about parrots, but never thought to ask:
"A quarter of the world's 352 species of parrots are at risk of extinction in their native habitats."

"Only two parrot species were native to the continental United States:" The Carolina Parakeet and the Thick-billed Parrot (still found in Mexico); both are now extinct due to habitat destruction and hunting. Populations of non-native feral parrots that live in the United States are either escaped pets or descendants of escapees.

Does Polly Want a Cracker?

Not all parrots eat the same thing in the wild. It depends on the specie, what it's drawn to, and what is up for grabs. Their natural diet is a smorgasbord of foods such as seeds, grains, nuts, fruits, nectar, pollen, flowers, bark, buds, roots, insects and invertebrates. "In general, palm nuts and nuts are their favorites."

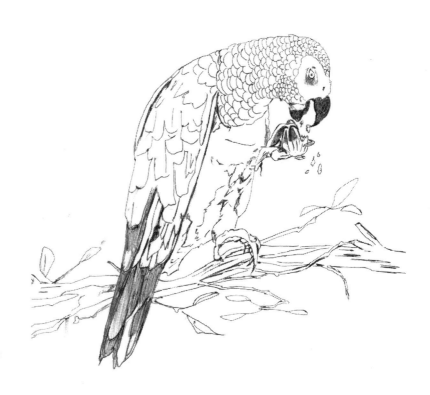

Like all wildlife, parrots have to hunt and work for their food: Their powerful claws are adept at tearing apart tough, fibrous husks from seeds and nuts. "Their extraordinary beak allows them to reach a supply of food unavailable to other birds. Only a bird with special adaptations and ingenuity can reach these feasts."

If you have a pet parrot, keep him occupied. Give him a job to do, such as separating shells from pistachio nuts, and removing tough peels from fruits and other plants that he might eat. This will result in a healthier, happier pet and companion.

Do All Parrots Mimic?
Only pet parrots mimic people and repeat phrases. The African Grey rocks!

When bringing home a new pet parrot, it is always wise to first consult with a vet about your bird's specific diet and other needs.

The Chipmunk

6 ounces frozen bananas - cut into ½-inch pieces
1 cup chocolate soy milk or 1% milk + 2 Tablespoons cocoa
2 rounded Tablespoons almonds
1 or 2 dates (seeds removed) diced in ¼-inch pieces

Place almonds in blender jar. Return lid and process until finely ground. Turn off blender and add rest of ingredients. Separate fruit with a sturdy plastic tool. Return lid and pulse in short bursts about 8 to 10 times. Turn off pulse button and process until smooth, a matter of seconds.

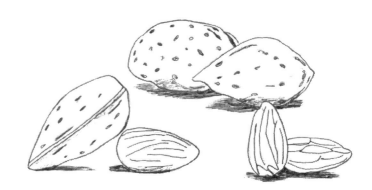

The truth is out. The **almond** we all love is really not a nut, but a seed from the fruit of the beautiful flowering almond tree. It is related to stone fruits such as the peach, apricot and cherry. Nutty as it seems, we eat the seed and throw away the fruit.

"The earliest varieties of almonds were found in China, carried by traders down the Silk Road to Greece, Turkey, and the Middle East." It wasn't until the 1700s that almond trees arrived in North America. They were brought over from Spain by the Franciscan Padres, who planted the trees in California. Today, California remains "the only place in North America where almonds are grown commercially."

Adding almonds to your diet is a great way to put variety into the meat and beans group without the saturated fats and cholesterol found in animal foods. Just one ounce of almonds offers six grams of good quality protein, significant amounts of fiber and vitamin E, plus "a unique blend of minerals that are beneficial to bone health." It doesn't hurt that they taste so good!

Almonds will retain their freshness if stored in a tight container in a cool dry place. For long periods of time, place in a ziplock bag and store in the freezer.

Chipmunks are related to squirrels and share some of the same characteristics. But while squirrels are arboreal (living in trees), chipmunks live in the ground. Only chipmunks have stripes on their heads and faces.

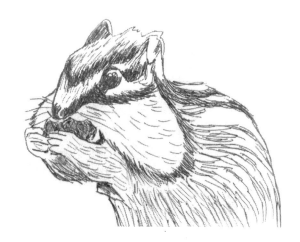

The most distinctive feature about chipmunks is their pouched cheeks, which have the amazing ability to carry lots of seeds and nuts for storing in their tunnels. You may be surprised to learn just "how much these cheek pouches can hold. Chipmunks have been observed carrying 27 hazelnuts, 31 corn kernels, 13 prune pits, 70 sunflower seeds, or 32 beechnuts in their cheek pouches at one time!"

Can you gather food like a chipmunk? Are you able to crack a nut with your teeth? Both of these features are physical adaptations that enable this perky little animal to live comfortably and secure in its home--that is until one of its predators, such as the weasel or snake, happens to come upon it.

Chipmunks play a significant role in the food web as prey for many animals and birds. Their tunneling activity plays an important role in the dispersion of seeds. "Any buried seeds that are not consumed have a better chance of germinating than those remaining on the surface. In this way, chipmunks assist in the spreading of shrubs, trees, and other plants." But quite possibly one of its biggest values is the pleasure it gives to hikers, campers, or anyone who happens to be lucky enough to see one.

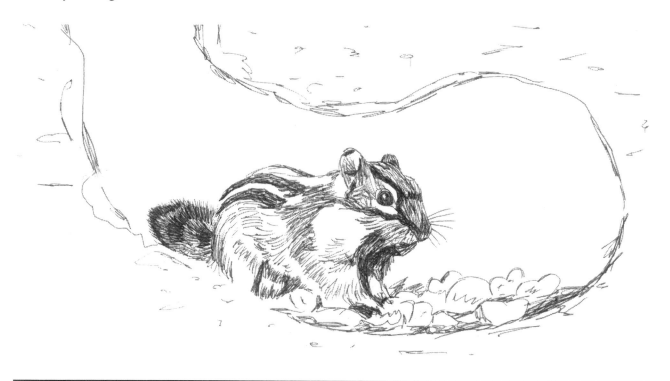

The Monkey

6 ounces frozen bananas - cut into ½-inch pieces
2 dates (seeds removed) diced in ¼-inch pieces
8 ounces vanilla soy milk or 2% milk
1 tsp. cream of coconut

Measure liquid into blender jar. Add
remaining ingredients. Separate fruit
with a sturdy plastic tool. Return lid
to blender jar. Pulse in short bursts
about 8 to 10 times. Turn off pulse
button and process until smooth, a
matter of seconds.

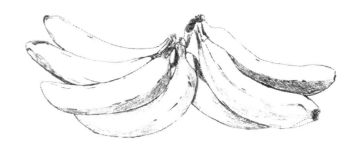

Many of us have heard the saying,
"Money doesn't grow on trees." Well, neither do bananas. They grow on very large herbs that
belong to a group of green plants with soft stems. Most flowers and grasses are also herbs.

Bananas are one of the most amazing foods on the planet. Besides all the health benefits, they
are always available, presently affordable, require no refrigeration, arrive in their own cheerful
packaging, and, best of all, taste delicious. That is why babies, children and adults all love
them.

Get ready for this: A serving size--a half cup--will give you 11% of the daily value requirement of potassium, making this fruit beneficial in lowering blood pressure. A half cup of
bananas also provides 10% of the daily value requirement of Vitamin C--very important for
growth and repair of body tissues.

Bananas feed the friendly bacteria in your digestive tract.

Bananas "have a higher carbohydrate content than most other fruits (by weight), making them
a good snack choice for endurance athletes." No wonder the monkey is so playful!

The Entertainer

Many species of "monkeys have developed prehensile tails" that work like another hand. This convenient adaptation enables them to grab a piece of fruit off a branch that would otherwise be out of reach.

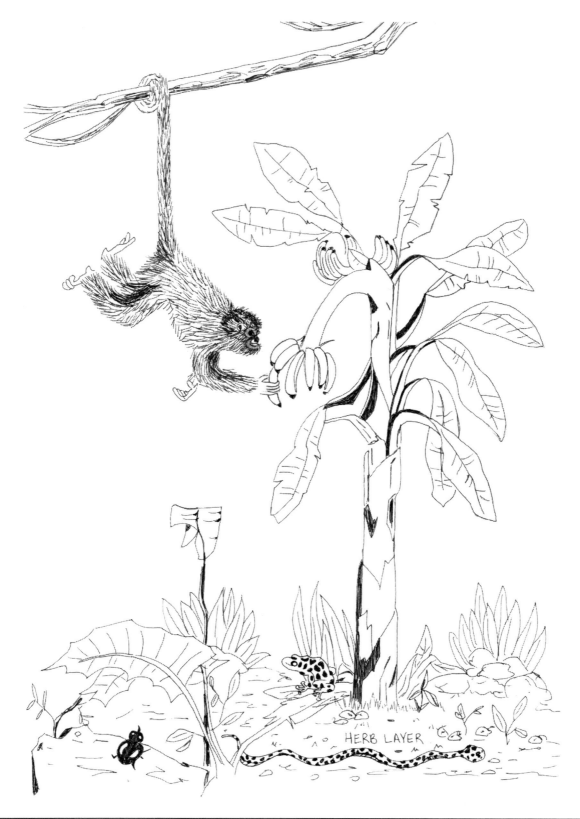

HERB LAYER

This not a choice for anyone allergic to peanuts. Try the chipmunk.

The Squirrel

6 ounces frozen bananas - cut into ½-inch pieces
8 ounces chocolate soy milk or 1% milk + 2 Tablespoons cocoa
2 Tablespoons peanut butter
1 or 2 dates (seeds removed) diced in ¼-inch pieces

Measure liquid into blender jar. Add rest of ingredients. Separate fruit with a sturdy plastic tool. Return lid to blender jar. Pulse in short bursts about 8 to 10 times. Turn off pulse button and process until smooth, a matter of seconds.

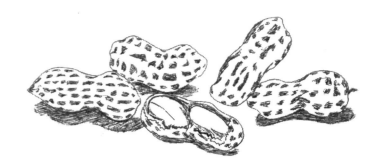

Did you know the peanut is not really a nut but a legume, a member of the pea family? And if you think that is nutty, there is more. The cashew is a seed and the acorn is a nut.

Peanuts originated in South America. "When Africans were brought to North America as slaves, peanuts came with them." Americans regarded the peanut as a poor man's food and fed them to the pigs. It wasn't until the Civil War that the peanut became a food source for humans, sustaining "the soldiers from both the North and South," when food was very scarce and the peanut was often the only thing around to eat.

Peanut butter had its beginning in 1890 when "a St. Louis physician developed the idea of packaging peanut paste for people with bad teeth." Today, "Americans eat three pounds of peanut butter per person every year--enough to coat the floor of the Grand Canyon."

Peanut butter is a good way to add protein to a meal or snack. Just "two Tablespoons--the amount in an average sandwich--provides about seven grams," plus several important vitamins and minerals. True, it does have a high fat content, but it is mostly monounsaturated fat, the healthy kind.

In this rich and delicious shake, peanut butter is combined with another favorite: chocolate. It's enough to make you go bananas!

Peanut Trivia: "Two former U.S. presidents were peanut farmers: Thomas Jefferson and Jimmy Carter."

Friend or foe--undecided? Then "take a good look at the next squirrel you see" and observe some of his features:

- Eyes placed at the sides of his head, better for spotting an enemy.

- Hind feet that can rotate 180 degrees, allowing sharp rear claws to hook onto bark when descending a tree.

- Forepaws adept at holding his food, enabling him to bite each scale on the pinecone, which holds his treasure--the two seeds that are rich in fats and nutrients.

- Large front teeth that are razor sharp and never stop growing.

- An incredible tail that acts as a parachute when descending a tree.

All of the above features are physical adaptations that make the grey squirrel so well suited for a life among the trees. Scientists believe he arrived about 63 million years ago, along with forests of seed- and nut-bearing trees.

The grey squirrel's behavior of burying acorns is not only beneficial to himself, providing food during the harder winter months, but also benefits the forest as well. His "good memory and keen sense of smell" enables him to retrieve his food, but there are times when he overlooks or forgets about it. Those unretrieved acorns often become new tree seedlings, helping to restore the hardwood forest.

Grey squirrels supplement their diet with fruit, leaf buds, bark, pine cone seeds, insects, and birds eggs, but acorns and hickory nuts are the main component of their diet, providing fat and carbohydrates for the more difficult months ahead. A squirrel's gnawing action on nuts is what keeps his front teeth sharp and short; this is very important for his survival.

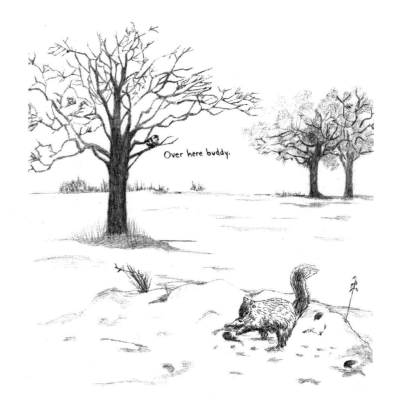

Over here buddy.

If you think you like squirrels a little better now, celebrate by eating a handful of nuts. They are good for you, too.

This shake is not recommended for young children.

Spunky Monkey

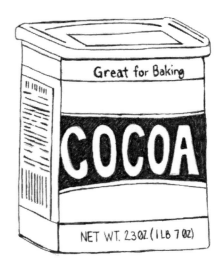

6 ounces frozen bananas cut into ½-inch pieces
2 Tablespoons decaffeinated espresso beans
1 cup chocolate soy milk or 1% milk + 2 Tablespoons cocoa
2 Tablespoons almonds
2 dates (seeds removed) diced in ¼-inch pieces

In blender jar, process almonds until finely ground. Turn off blender. Add liquid, fruit, cocoa (if using), and espresso beans. Separate fruit with a sturdy plastic tool. Return lid and pulse in short bursts about 8 to 10 times. Turn off pulse button and process until smooth, a matter of seconds.

I love the combination of coffee and chocolate in this delicious shake. In moderation, both are now considered good for you.

"**Chocolate** and **cocoa powder** are derived from beans (or seeds) that contain hefty quantities of natural antioxidants called flavonoids." Similar flavonoids can be found in other foods, such as cranberries, apples, tea, and red wine.

Great news for chocoholics: "Just 1/4 ounce or 30 calories a day of dark chocolate has been linked to lower blood pressure without causing weight gain." So go ahead--delight in a bite!

Did you know that chocolate grows naturally on trees in the rainforest understory? In actuality, it is encased in football-shaped pods (or fruit) that grow directly out of the trunk and branches.

When mature, "each pod holds about 30 to 50 cocoa seeds, enough to make about seven milk chocolate bars or two dark chocolate bars."

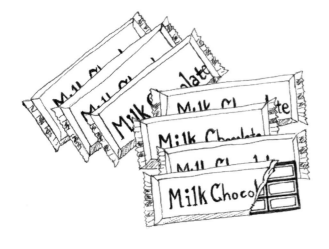

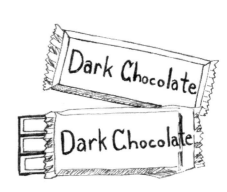

Many animals and birds that live in the rainforest, such as the monkey and toucan, have symbiotic relationships with understory trees: They enjoy the sweet pulp from the cocoa pods, but dislike the bitter taste of the seeds, the real treasure. They spit them out, spreading them on to the forest floor; this results in a new generation of trees.

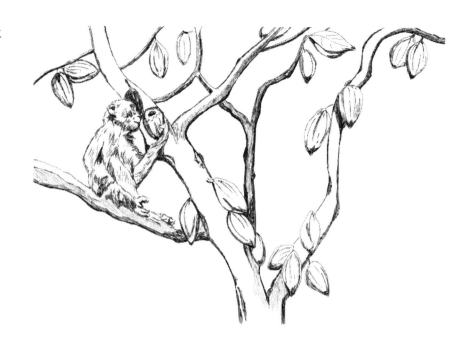

"A tiny fly no bigger than the head of a pin is responsible for the world's supply of chocolate."

— Allen Young

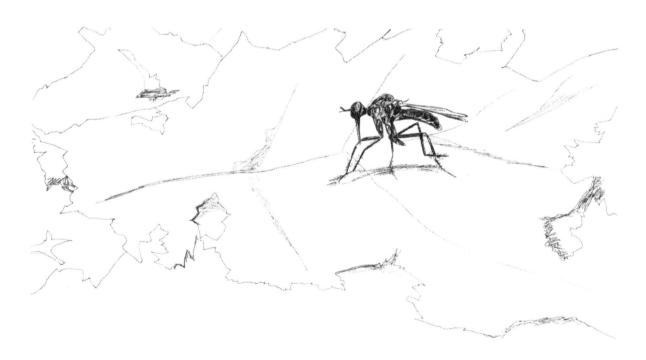

In the wild, cocoa trees are "pollinated by tiny flies called midges, which thrive in the decaying leaf litter of the rainforest floor." The tiny flowers of the cocoa tree "grow directly on the trunk and lower branches." These flowers are "complicated in design, and the midge is the only animal that can work its way through the flower."

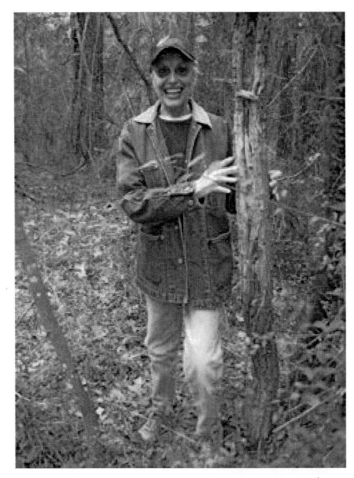

Author enjoying a walk at the Houston Arboretum & Nature Center - 2010

CHAPTER 5

It's a Green Thing

A Return to Nature

Walk Gently With the Creatures

Partying With the Creatures

Make A Shake Sleepover and Naturalist Walk

Stump the Naturalist - Game 1

Stump the Naturalist - Game 2

Wildlife Birthday Party

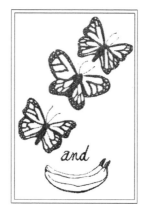

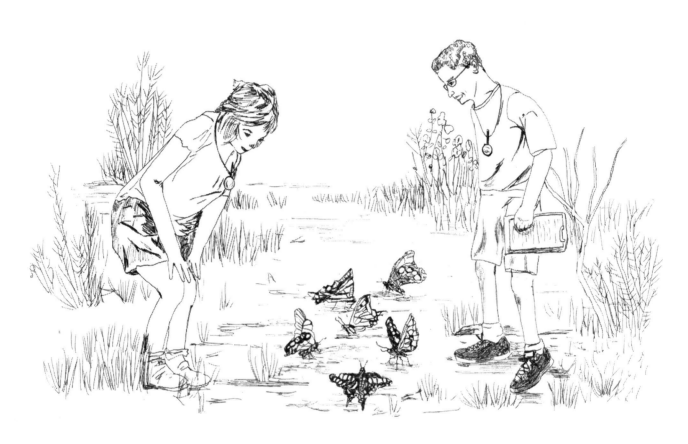

"A sense of wonder and joy in nature should be at the very center of ecological literacy."

- Richard Louv

A Return to Nature

Today, many of America's youth are disconnected from nature. They have never spent time exploring the outdoors. They have never seen a turtle or caterpillar. Many are overbooked with indoor activites. They live in a world where technology has overtaken their lives. Whatever the reason for the disconnect, we need to have our children return to nature.

Why? Children must have contact and experience with the natural world if they are to become responsible stewards of the planet. The most important reason may simply be that children love to explore. It is a natural healthy instinct that ought to be encouraged. Evidence has shown direct contact with nature is vital to the emotional and physical health of our youth. Children who bond with nature at a young age are rewarded with happy, carefree memories of physical interaction and discovery that cannot be replicated on our video screens, Xboxes or computers. Time spent on video and games, means less time for "homework, exercising or exploring."

What can replace the excitement of what you thought to be a rock turned out to be a snapping turtle flaunting its disguise? Or accidentally coming upon a coral snake in its natural habitat? Viewing a group of swallowtail butterflies busily getting sustenance from a mud hole?

Many of us have heard calls from doctors, the government, and educators about the importance of participating in age-appropriate moderate to vigorous physical activity. We are being asked to do this most days of the week in addition to our daily routine. A one- to two-mile walk at a nature preserve or park is one way to accomplish this goal while having fun and enjoying the natural beauty and allure of your surroundings.

Walk Gently with the Creatures

When you enter a forest, prairie, park or nature preserve, you will most likely come in contact with a community of animals that you may never see. Yet they could be close by, hidden in the hollow of a tree, a burrow, or beneath a pile of leaves, quite possibly asleep. We call these animals nocturnal. As you explore their habitat, be aware that you are entering the homes of many different creatures. Walk gently. Respect their right to rest and seek shelter.

The best way to explore nature is quietly. The natives who lived before us were experts at this; they totally depended on the land for their survival. They often called upon their keen observation skills and highly developed senses to assist them with their tracking. I have been witness to many missed opportunities to view wildlife, though unintentional, simply because of sudden noise. One time I spotted a beautiful bronze frog perched on a log with only its profile in view, so still and glistening it looked like a piece of sculpture. Another time I caught a glimpse of the colorful coral snake, relatively shy and not commonly spotted, that took shelter in the brush nearby.

The next time you are out and about, remember those who walked before you. You are certain to have a much better time if you do.

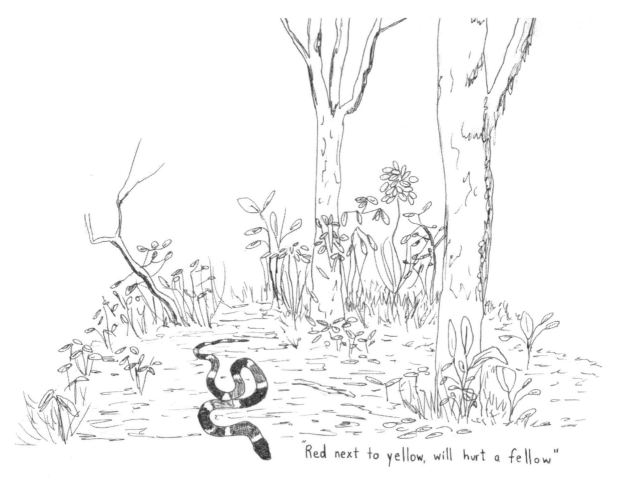

"Red next to yellow, will hurt a fellow"

*This phrase is often used to differentiate the coral snake (a venomous snake) from the milk snake that has similar colored bands, but is not harmful.

Partying With the Creatures

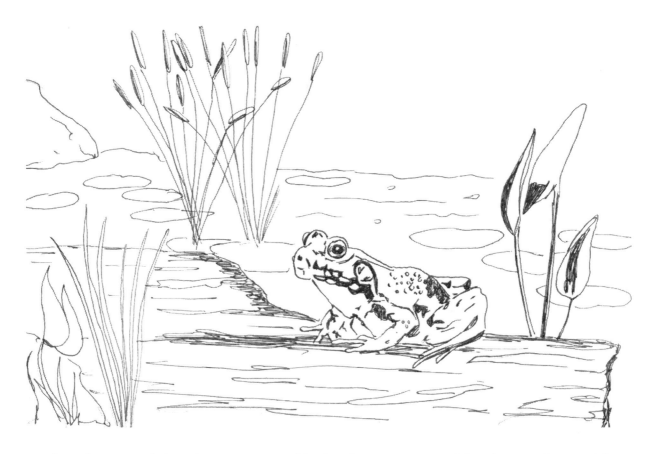

Now that Planet Earth is going green, consider having your next celebration outdoors with a nature theme. It doesn't have to be an elaborate or time-consuming affair. Often, the simplest parties turn out to be the most successful.

Here are two down-to-earth parties that enable children to have direct contact with nature. They require a little ingenuity, but are well worth the effort. Children get in plenty of exercise, a chance to explore, and a healthy dose of fun. Chaperones enjoy it, too.

The "Make a Shake Sleepover & Naturalist Walk" is designed for a small group ages nine to adult. This is an opportunity for children to be creative and exhibit organizational skills. The party begins in the home with a sleepover, and ends outdoors. In the evening, children and adults participate in the fun and challenging game of *Stump the Naturalist,* pages 70-71, created just for this party.

"The Wildlife Birthday Party" is a scavenger hunt suitable for children ages seven to adult. Older children and adults enjoy this as much as the younger children, making it appropriate for scouts and other groups. This takes place entirely out of doors, in a park or forest, and ends with a picnic lunch. Although a good bit of organization is required here, there is really little fuss or muss—a winner every time!

Make a Shake Sleepover and Naturalist Walk

This party begins in the evening with a "green hour" of fun. Children (ages 9 and up), assume the role of naturalists while the facilitator (older sibling or parent) lead the group in a very challenging and entertaining game of: *Stump the Naturalist* (pages 70 and 71). It is suggested that you play no longer than an hour with a break in between, possibly for refreshments or birthday cake, if appropriate.

The following morning each child will *"Make a Shake"* for breakfast. I recommend that you and your child select three different shakes from the "Forest Shake Index" (page 25) and print out in duplicates or more, if needed. Keep in mind that each of these shakes will serve one to two children. Have all the shake ingredients ready, along with an appropriate little party gift. Example: The Chipmunk - bag of nuts; The Bee - jar of honey; The Bat - Agave Nectar. Have your child decorate little paper sacks with a corresponding animal theme in which to carry home their gifts.

I recommend having finger sandwiches, such as pimento cheese or tuna salad, to eat with the shakes. These can be prepared the day before. After breakfast, the children will don their magnifying glasses as the "green team" gets ready for the naturalist walk. If you are planning a long outing, you may want to give each child and adult water and a small bag of trail mix to take along.

Plan a hike where children can have fun and explore in a natural setting. Most kids love to see frogs, turtles, snakes and insects. If the weather is nice, and you know of a large pond or riparian area, consider going there. The most important thing is to allow the children to safely explore and investigate without any directed activity. You will be amazed at what they will discover.

Children will be very excited. You will want to lay a few ground rules before you start out. Visit page 64, "Walk Gently with the Creatures," for a few good tips on viewing wildlife. Take a knowledgeable person with you to answer a few questions or act as a guide. Many nature centers have guides who will do this for a fee, if you wish.

After the hike children will be hungry and ready for lunch. Think pizza. The party ends at the house where the young naturalists gather their belongings and say goodbye.

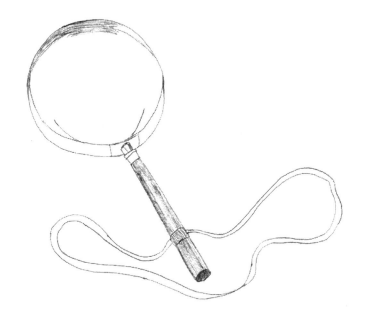

If you are planning this sleepover as a birthday party, you may want to send out invitations. An older sibling or parent can do this on the computer or by hand. Have your child pick an appropriate theme, for example: woodpecker, raccoon, pond, etc. Specify location and pick-up time.

Now for the game. This is how it works: Children are seated at a table. A parent or older sibling will hand each child a magnifying lens as they assume the role of "naturalist." Explain that you will be trying to stump them with your questions. Select a quitting time before you begin.

Starting clockwise, the leader will ask one of the naturalists to choose any number from 1 to 30. The leader will then read that participant the corresponding question from the "Stump the Naturalist" list. The participant will attempt to answer that question. If the answer is correct, leader will quack the duck, and record the number and designated score under the child's name. If the participant is unable to answer the question, the leader will have stumped the naturalist and the frog will ribbit. Other children can then have a chance to respond to the question, score points, or move on to the next player. Keep it light! Discussion is encouraged. Whoever has the highest score wins the game.

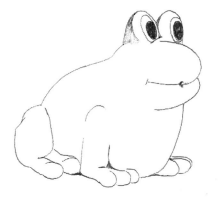

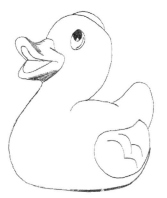

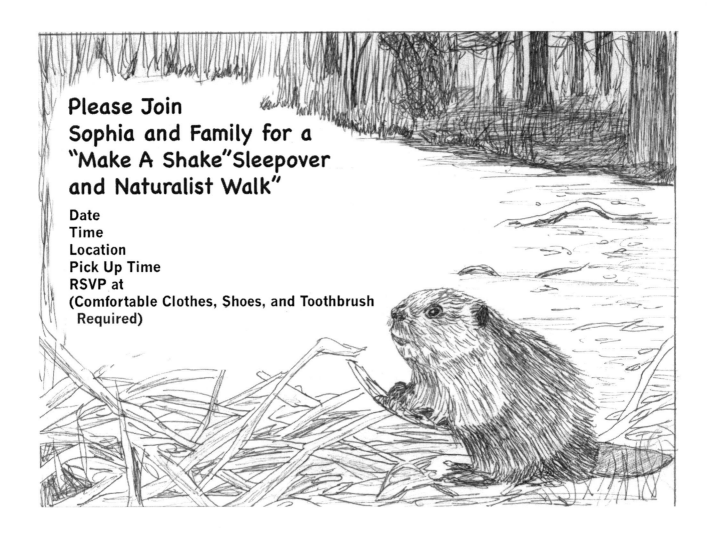

**Please Join
Sophia and Family for a
"Make A Shake"Sleepover
and Naturalist Walk"**

Date
Time
Location
Pick Up Time
RSVP at
(Comfortable Clothes, Shoes, and Toothbrush
   Required)

Small plastic magnifying lens are inexpensive and usually available at most nature shops. Children will take the lens on their morning walk, then home as a souvenir from the party. These lenses can be purchased at most nature shops for around five dollars.

A small toy duck that quacks and a frog that ribbits adds a little element of fun to the game. These are available at most neighborhood toy stores.

On pages 74 and 75 you will find a second set of "Stump the Naturalist" questions to be played at another time, straight from your book. This is a great thing to do in the evenings on family vacations or weekend outings, and there is so little to pack. Best of all, adults like it, too. Just don't forget the frog and the duck!

Stump the Naturalist - Ages Nine to Adult

Animal is used to imply any creature, such as: bird, insect, or snake.

1. What animal is our closet living relative? Chimpanzee.   5

2. Name two ways in which the wind affects ecosystems. Pollination, seed dispersal, soil erosion, temperature change.   10

3. What bird can hover in space like a helicopter? Hummingbird.   5

4. "Red next to yellow can hurt a fellow," applies to what snake? Coral snake.   **10**

5. How do squirrels contribute to the environment? By burying acorns and nuts that often turn into new tree seedlings.   5

6. What marine animal has survived the extinction of the dinosaur and is still present in the world's oceans today? Marine turtles.   **15**

7. What is the primary purpose of a flower? Reproduction - produce seed.   **8**

8. Name five things that may cause a tree to fall down? Fire, man, disease, wind, lightning.   5

9. Animals and humans that eat both plant and animal food are called?   Omnivores.   **8**

10. Why do animals migrate? Weather, food, and to reproduce.   5

11. Name four ways in which trees are beneficial to the environment? Filter out pollutants from the air, take in carbon dioxide, pump out oxygen, provide shelter, food, and humidity; tree roots prevent soil erosion.   **8**

12. How do bats in North America help the environment? They consume over 600 insects an hour, including mosquitos.   5

13. What creature is the most important pollinator of the world's food crops?   European honeybee.   **10**

14. The home or address of a plant or animal is called a…?   Habitat.   5

15. Name the only great ape found in Asia. The Orangutan.   **10**

16. What do birds and turtles have in common? Both have beaks.   **15**

17. Animals like the squirrel that are active during the day and sleep at night, are called? Diurnal—the same applies to humans.   **10**

18. Name one way in which animals and birds help plants distribute their seed? By transporting seed to new locations in their feathers or fur; by depositing undigested seed in their droppings at new locations.   **8**

19. Who is the most important bird pollinator of wildflowers in the continental United States? The Hummingbird.   **10**

20. As a naturalist on an expedition, name four things you might want to bring along? Food, water, first aid kit, camera, magnifying glass, buddy, journal.   **5**

21. What came first, the chicken or the egg? The egg came first, because birds are descendants of egg-laying reptiles.   **15**

22. What is the ecological role of fungi (mushrooms) and bacteria? Decomposer   **8**

23. Plants that capture energy from the sun to make food are called? Producers.   **8**

24. Animals like the rabbit that eat only plants are called? Herbivores.   **8**

25. If Daddy-longlegs is not a spider, and spins no web, what is it? A Harvestman, closely related to mites. Two of its legs act as antennas that allow them to feel, smell and taste.   **15**

26. What bird is clumsy on land and cannot fly? The penguin.   **5**

27. Characteristics that enable animals to do certain things and survive in their environment are called?   Adaptations.   **10**

28. The polar bear is listed as threatened under the Endangered Species Act; why? The effects of climate change on its Arctic Ocean ice habitat.   **8**

29. Name the only mammal that can fly. Bat   **8**

30. Name four things that all living things need to survive. Food, water, shelter, space.   **5**

Vermont 2005 - Author examining fungi on family vacation.

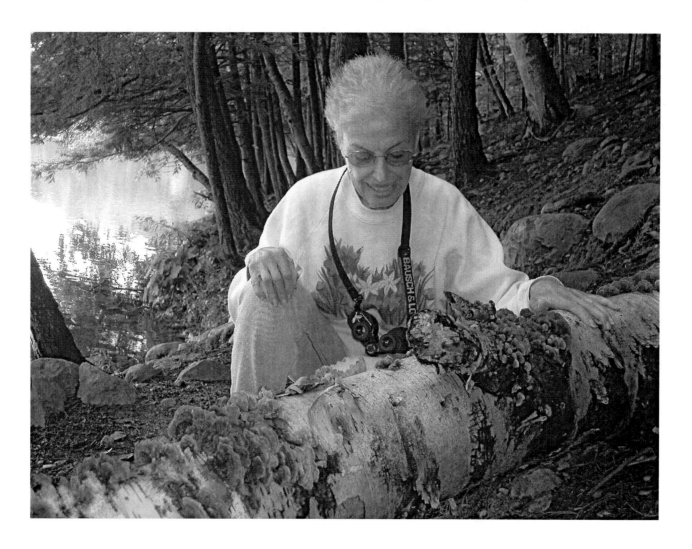

"Look deep into nature, and then you will understand everything better."
—Albert Einstein

Stump the Naturalist - Part 2

"Animal" is used to imply any creature, such as: mammal, bird, insect, or snake.

1. What group of animals lay eggs in water and typically have four limbs? Amphibians.   8

2. How do rainforests help control the earth's climate? Storing carbon dioxide and recycling rain fall when it evaporates.   15

3. Name the largest animal on earth? Blue whale.   15

4. Animals that nurse their young are called? Mammals.   8

5. What is the scientific name for all living things? Organism.   5

6. When a tadpole enters the adult stage to become a frog, it has completed its…? Metamorphosis.   10

7. Electricity that is powered by the sun is called? Solar energy.   10

8. Animals that eat only meat are called? Carnivores.   5

9. In the winter months, what do some animals do to conserve energy when food is scarce? Hibernate.   8

10. What very famous naturalist said, "When one tugs at a single thing in nature, he finds it attached to the rest of the world."   John Muir.   15

11. Why does the Monarch butterfly deposit her eggs on the milkweed plant? It is the only plant her offspring will eat.   10

12. What ecosystem are you likely to see lots of frogs? Wetlands and ponds.   5

13. An organism's role or job in an ecosystem is called a? Niche.   10

14. What ecosystem is home to grasshoppers, gophers, wildflowers, and many birds? Prairie (meadow).   5

15. Name two valuable products that come from the bee? Honey and bees wax.   8

16. Name the only mammal with a shell. Armadillo has a shell much like a turtle.   **8**

17. Name three simple ways in which we can help the environment? 1 - recycle, 2 - take our own bags to stores to carry home groceries and other products, 3 - turn off equipment and lights when not in use, 4 - Run the dishwasher only when full.   **15**

18. What was Al Gore's film *An Inconvenient Truth* about? Global warming.   **8**

19. Who is the largest carnivore on land? Polar bear.   **10**

20. Features that enable woodpeckers to hammer holes in trees in order to obtain food or make a home are called? Physical adaptations.   **10**

21. The name "Masked Bandit" describes what well known animal? Raccoon.   **5**

22. What do a raccoon and polar bear have in common? Both like to go fishing and both have the same walking pattern.   **8**

23. All food chains begin with? Energy from the sun.   **5**

24. Why do mosquitos bite? Only the pregnant female bites; she needs a high protein meal in order for her eggs to develop properly.   **15**

25. Name the only lizard that can swim in the oceans. Marine Iguana of the Galapagos.   **15**

26. What butterfly is known for its lengthy migration? Monarch.   **5**

27. What does the kangaroo and opossum have in common? Both are marsupial, meaning they carry their young in a pouch.   **10**

28. The first environmental president in the United States was? Theodore Roosevelt.   **10**

29. Why do carnivorous plants like the Venus Fly Trap eat insects? Most carnivorous plants live in nutrient-poor habitats. "Enriching their diets with nitrogen captured from animals help them thrive."   **15**

30. What plant is foraged more by wildlife than any other plant?   Grass.   **8**

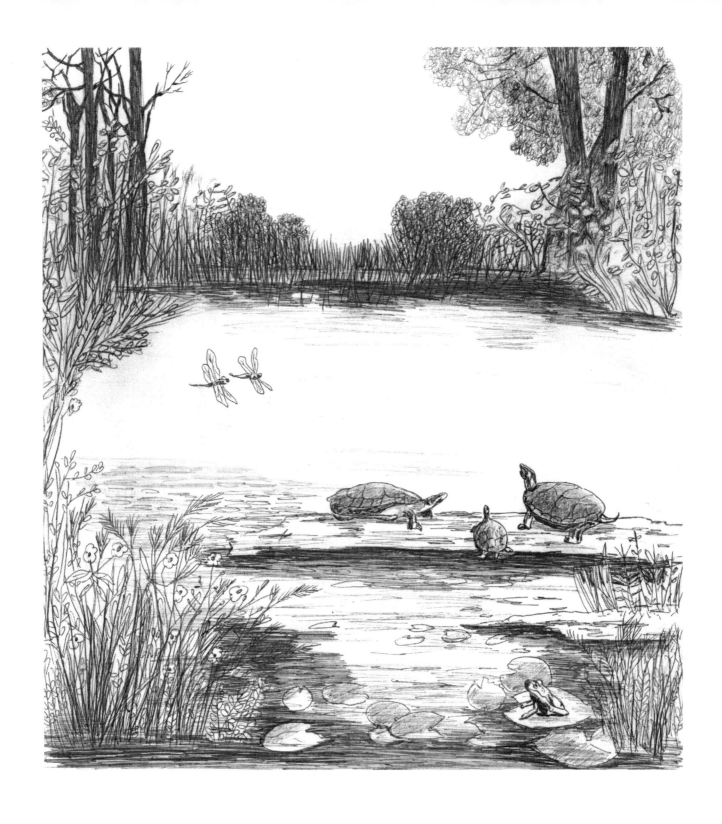

"Come forth into the light of things. Let nature be your teacher."

— William Wordsworth

Wildlife Birthday Party

For this party you will lead children on a scavenger hunt through a forest or park. You will need two responsible and enthusiastic adults to lead a group of 10 children.

Most forests and parks have well-marked trails and maps for hiking. You will want to stake it out first, looking for evidence of where wildlife has been. If you are reluctant to do this, many nature centers have naturalists who will lead a group for you for a fee. Plan a picnic close by.

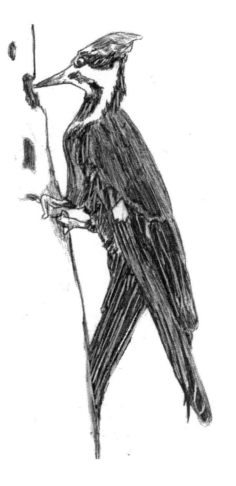

It's A Wildlife Birthday Party!

Please Join Aden for a Hike and Picnic Lunch.

Date

Time

Location

Pick Up Time and Location

RSVP at

Comfortable Clothes and Shoes Required

Invitations - Involve the Family:

Allow your child to select an animal or other appropriate theme. Older siblings can design the invitation on a computer. Detail arrival and pickup time, location, and note that lunch or refreshments will follow. I recommend a mid-morning hike when children are energetic and ready to be outdoors.

What you will need:

Backpack for leader only, containing:

- 2 maps of the trails - one for each adult

- Mosquito repellent

- First aid kit

- 10 small plastic magnifying lenses for each child to wear and keep

- 10 small pencils

- 10 wildlife checklists - <u>customized to the locality</u> - example, page 79

- A small rubber stamp of a tree and ink pad - optional

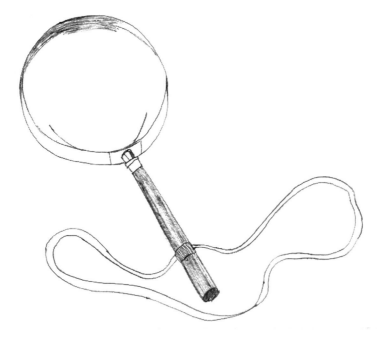

These supplies can be purchased at most nature shops and nature centers.
They are inexpensive, and you can add whatever you like to your theme. Keep it simple.

SCAVENGER HUNT CHECKLIST
Put a checkmark beside each wildlife clue you find.

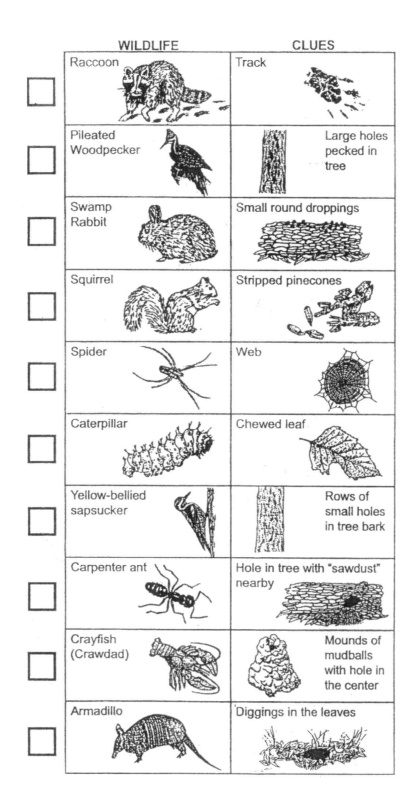

	WILDLIFE		CLUES	
☐	Raccoon		Track	
☐	Pileated Woodpecker		Large holes pecked in tree	
☐	Swamp Rabbit		Small round droppings	
☐	Squirrel		Stripped pinecones	
☐	Spider		Web	
☐	Caterpillar		Chewed leaf	
☐	Yellow-bellied sapsucker		Rows of small holes in tree bark	
☐	Carpenter ant		Hole in tree with "sawdust" nearby	
☐	Crayfish (Crawdad)		Mounds of mudballs with hole in the center	
☐	Armadillo		Diggings in the leaves	

*Checklist: Customized at the Houston Arboretum & Nature Center for activities and birthday parties

Begin by assembling the group and a giving brief orientation:

Children will be very excited. Lay a few ground rules by telling children to be respectful of the animals that live there; that they should be orderly while following the leader and to stay on the trails. Chaperone(s) will follow in the rear.

Leader will begin by telling the children they are: forest or park detectives, who will be hunting for animal evidence, just like real detectives do when attempting to solve a case.

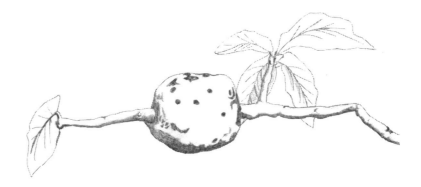

Leader will give each child a:

- Wildlife checklist

- Pencil

- Naturalist magnifying lens

Upon completion of the hike, the leader will stamp each child's hand with a tree stamp, proclaiming them "Forest or Park Detectives." Children will take their checklists, magnifying lens, and memories home.

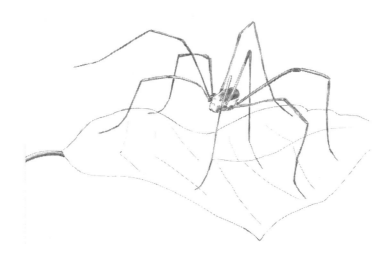

CHAPTER **6**

For the Love of It

Just for the love of it, I have included several of my family's favorite recipes. Some date back to the 80s; others came much later. All are because someone, or something, inspired me to create them. They are incredibly nourishing, delicious, and fun to prepare.

It is my hope that these recipes might kindle a passion within you, empowering you as you continue down the road best taken—the one that leads to vitality and optimum health.

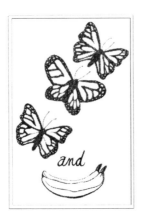

*Vegan

Back in the eighties when oat bran was touted as a cholesterol healthy food, muffins began popping up everywhere. This led me to create my own version—a healthy quick breakfast that my husband could down along with his coffee as he raced out the door. One could accurately say this was a labor of love. It still is today. They are especially popular with the rest of my family during our yearly trip to the Texas Hill Country, when all of us are ready to head out the door, eager to begin our morning hikes.

Because I love to give these muffins for gifts, I often make an extra batch for the freezer. Why not? I have everything out, and who wouldn't care for an exceptional, healthy, homemade muffin?

Have you seen those cute little food bags and boxes that are now available at specialty stores? They beg to be taken home.

One's a Meal Muffins

Makes 12 muffins

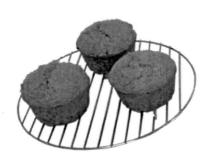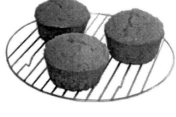

1/4 cup canola oil
1/2 cup coconut juice
1/3 cup pure honey
1 large egg*
1 cup vanilla soy milk
1/4 teaspoon vanilla
1cup golden raisins

1 cup whole wheat pastry flour
1 teaspoon baking soda
1/2 teaspoon salt
1 cup quick cooking rolled oats
1/2 cup - minus 1 Tablespoon wheat bran
1/2 cup - minus 1 Tablespoon oat bran
1/2 cup walnut or pecan pieces- optional

Preheat oven 325 degrees.

Simmer raisins in coconut juice until softened. Allow to cool.

In a large mixing bowl, mix together pastry flour, baking soda, and salt. Stir in rest of the dry ingredients, blending all together.

Into blender jar, place raisins and coconut juice mixture. Add honey, egg, vanilla soy, canola oil, and vanilla. On the "chop" button, process until well blended, a matter of seconds.

Add wet ingredients to the dry. Follow with the nuts. With a wooden spoon, mix all ingredients together until no trace of flour remains. **Do not beat.** Allow to set 5 minutes before filling pans.

Pour mixture into a lightly oiled muffin pan that yields 12. Bake about 23 to 25 minutes, or until tested clean. Remove pan from oven, and place on a rack to cool, about 10 minutes.

Remove muffins from pan by gently loosening sides with a dinner knife. Muffins will slide out nicely. Place on rack until completely cooled.

Substitutions:

Vanilla soy milk - buttermilk to which you would add 1/4 teaspoon vanilla.

Whole wheat pastry flour - whole wheat flour or regular all-purpose flour.

Raisins - Be creative and have fun. I recently made a batch using 3/4 cups dried cranberries, and 1/4 cup diced crystalized ginger that got raves.

*Eggs 101: If you are concerned about cholesterol, use1 large omega 3 fortified egg, or 1/4 cup egg substitute, or 2 large egg whites.

Chef's Tips:

Pastry flour imparts a more delicate texture to breads and muffins.

You can either drink (it is very nourishing) or freeze the remaining coconut juice in 4-ounce increments for later use.

One day while shopping at the neighborhood supermarket, I came upon an incredible buy on some beautiful wild fish—fresh king salmon. Now, that turns me on! Although I didn't have a clue as to what I would do with all the filets I bought that day, there were two things I did know: I had a freezer, and salmon is way up there on the list of healthy foods. Although I do buy farm-raised fish, I prefer to eat the wild whenever I can, because I know it has eaten directly from the food chain and therefore has a nice concentration of those important DHA Omega 3 fish oils we have heard so much about.*

Salmon is such a versatile fish. It did not take me long to come up with a couple ideas for my beautiful filets. My salmon patties are an updated version of those that were popular in the 50s, but I believe you will find these to be even more delicious. When there are children present, I make a point of serving them with mashed potatoes and green beans—adults not minding this accommodation.

*The omega 3 fatty acids that are found in wild fish actually originate from algae—a microscopic plant at the base of the marine food chain.

Scrumptious Salmon Patties

Makes 4 large patties

1 pound salmon filet
1/4 cup extra virgin olive oil
2 cloves, finely diced garlic
1/3 cup finely diced onion
1/4 teaspoon lite Creole seasoning
1/3 cup finely diced red bell pepper
Extra bread crumbs for dredging
1 large egg or egg substitute
1/4 cup bread crumbs
1 1/2 Tablespoons fresh lemon juice
Dash of tabasco sauce - optional

Preheat oven to 400 degrees. Lightly coat a 15-inch piece of foil with non-stick cooking spray. Cut salmon filet in half. Place salmon skin side down on coated side of foil. Completely cover salmon with both sides of foil, leaving ends open to vent. Place foil packet on cookie sheet and slide in oven for about 5 to 8 minutes. Remove salmon from oven and carefully open package. Salmon will be undercooked. Allow to cool a few minutes.

Transfer salmon to work bowl, along with juices. Discard skin and foil. Flake salmon with fork into small pieces. With your hands, gently toss garlic, bell pepper, onion and seasonings into the flaked salmon. Gradually toss in the bread crumbs, egg, and lemon juice until all ingredients are well incorporated. Taste and adjust seasonings accordingly.

Coat a platter with the extra bread crumbs. Divide salmon mixture into four, 4-inch patties and generously dredge each side with the crumbs. Season both sides lightly with Creole seasoning.

Cover a large skillet with the olive oil. When oil comes to temperature on medium hot, sauté patties three minutes on each side or until lightly browned. Serve while hot.

Chef's Tip: You can make ahead of time by covering the patties with foil and refrigerating a few hours or overnight. Just bring to room temperature about an hour before cooking time.

A bad weather forecast one evening altered my plans. Dinner out became dinner in. I have always said, "Give me a lemon, garlic, and an onion, and I am in business." I am one that loves the spontaneity and challenge of getting in the kitchen and using whatever is around. With a lime replacing the lemon, shrimp in the freezer—a few key ingredients waiting—how could I go wrong? I didn't! This was a keeper. Later that evening I revised the recipe to serve four. I make this dish often now, serving it with a few steamed broccoli florets on the side. A green salad completes this exceptional meal.

Shrimp Linguini with Cilantro Citrus

Serves 4

10 ounces medium/large shrimp, peeled and deveined
4 large cloves garlic, diced
1/8 to 1/4 teaspoon red pepper flakes
3 Tablespoons + 1 teaspoon fresh lime juice

Marinate the above ingredients in refrigerator for 1 hour.

1/3 cup extra virgin olive oil
1 1/4 pounds fresh plum tomatoes
3/4 cup diced red onion
4 large cloves garlic, diced
1/4 to 1/2 teaspoon salt
Approximately 1/2 cup diced cilantro leaves
8 ounces whole wheat linguine cooked al dente

Discard center core and most of the seeds in tomatoes. Dice.

Heat olive oil in a medium-size skillet. When oil comes to temperature, add onion, garlic, tomatoes and salt. Cook over medium-low heat until sauce is thick but not dry, about 10 minutes.

Add shrimp and marinade to skillet. Continue cooking a couple of minutes, stirring, until shrimp turn pink and curls. Do not overcook. Taste sauce and correct seasonings. Turn off heat and stir in cilantro. Allow sauce to sit a few minutes as you drain and plate the pasta. Distribute sauce and shrimp over the pasta and serve immediately.

Chef's Tip: Food processors work well on tomatoes. Do not puree.

As a way of keeping our cholesterol in check, I try to serve a few vegan meals for dinner each week. At first this met with opposition from my husband, a carnivore at heart. But, after considerable prodding on the merits of my reasoning, he finally acquiesced. This is hardly punishment! Still, whenever I come up with a vegan meal that he really likes—well, I feel like dancing.

On a family vacation in Vermont, I tried out this recipe for marinara sauce. My grandson, 12 years old at the time and a budding chef himself, assisted me. He chiffonade the basil, and we each took a turn at stirring the sauce; there is something therapeutic about stirring marinara sauce with your grandchild.

When we returned home, I learned that Jared put his personal touch on the recipe, using oregano instead of the basil. (He tried to sell me on oregano when we were in Vermont.) I also discovered that my daughter-in-law made it for her family who were visiting from Costa Rica. Maria said she forgot to add the wine to the sauce, "But it was still very delicious."

Fresh Marinara Sauce

Makes 3 1/2 cups - 6 to 7 as a main course

1/3 cup extra virgin olive oil
2 1/2 pounds fresh plum tomatoes
1/3 cup diced onion
6 to 7 large cloves garlic, diced
10 large chiffonade basil leaves
1/8 teaspoon cayenne pepper
1/4 to 1/2 teaspoon salt
1 1/2 Tablespoons tomato paste
1 Tablespoon of wine, preferably white

Discard center core and most of the seeds in tomatoes. Dice.

Place olive oil in medium-size skillet. Add all ingredients except basil. Simmer over low heat about 20 to 30 minutes (stirring occasionally) until sauce is thick, but not dry. Correct seasonings and turn off heat. Stir in basil.

Serve over your favorite pasta, preferably whole wheat

A green salad is the perfect accompaniment for this delicious meal.

Can be eaten hot or cold. Freezes well.

Chef's Tip: A food processor works well for dicing tomatoes. Pulse for even texture.

One day while shopping in the produce aisle for vegetables, I came across an apple green, pear-shaped type of squash that I had never seen before. They were very nice looking, free of blemishes, and all individually wrapped in plastic. What's more, they were cheap. Intrigued, I put a few in my grocery cart.

Later that day while preparing my vegetables, I decided to try these new little guys in a soup I was making. The next day (I like soup best the second day) my son Bob, whom I had invited for dinner along with his then girlfriend Maria, did not fail to notice that something new had been added to the soup. (Families don't let you get away with a thing!) When I told them about the interesting little squash I had discovered in the grocery store, Maria told us that Chayote (chee oh tay) is frequently used in soup in Costa Rica, her native country—often as the main ingredient. When Maria's family came to visit, I served this very same soup as a welcoming gesture. Seven months later, Bob and Maria were married. This time we had champagne.

Chayote Vegetable Soup with Beef

Makes 3 1/2 quarts

1 1/2 pounds beef shank bone with a good amount of meat and marrow*
3/4 cup dried cannellini* or great northern beans - rinsed
1/2 cup uncooked barley - rinsed
1 large onion - diced
1 medium Chayote squash - seeds removed, cut in 1-inch pieces
4 large carrots - peeled and cut into ½-inch pieces
2 large stocks celery - cut into ½-inch pieces
7 ounces green beans - trimmed and cut into 1-inch pieces
1/3 cup diced parsley, flat leaf variety preferred
1 14.5 ounce can diced tomatoes with liquid
2 Tablespoons chicken bouillon base of good quality
1/4 teaspoon salt
1/4 to 1/2 teaspoon black pepper
2 1/2 quarts water

Trim meat of surrounding fat. Place bone with meat and marrow in a 5 or 6 quart soup pot. Add water. Cover pot and bring to a boil.

Skim top of broth. With lid off, on medium heat, allow broth to reduce a little to concentrate flavor, about 30 minutes.

Add beans and barley. Cover pot and simmer 1 1/2 hours.

Remove meat and bone from pot, discarding the connective tissue. Cut meat in little chunks. Remove marrow from bone and mash with a fork. Discard bone. Return meat and marrow to pot. Continue simmering until meat and beans are almost tender.

Add onion, celery, carrots, green beans, chayote squash, tomatoes, bullion base and black pepper. Simmer about 30 minutes longer or until meat is fork tender and vegetables are done.

Taste and correct seasonings. (Soup is not meant to be spicy.) Add parsley and simmer 5 minutes longer to meld flavors.

When finished, soup should coat a spoon. To thicken, simply remove lid and simmer a little longer. Soup will also thicken overnight.

*It is best to soak cannellini beans a few hours or overnight to shorten cooking time.

*If cholesterol is a concern, you may want to discard the marrow along with the bones. Soup will still retain a good bit of flavor.

Chef's Tips: Bullion base + tasting are key here. My favorite brand is: Better Than Bullion Reduced Sodium Chicken Base.

Soup is equally delicious without the squash. Just add more of the other vegetables to make up the difference.

When the temperature begins to hover near forty, some brave souls grab their parkas and skis—others head out for warmer climates; many are happy to stay home with a book, eager to watch the next game on TV. I get out my stepladder and reach for my soup pot. On chilly days this soup pot has comforted a lot of people; young and old, well and ill.

One of the above was a cousin who was home recuperating from a serious surgery. Though I'm unsure of the role my soup played there, she made a complete recovery. This cousin is an extra-ordinary cook, so when she asked for the recipe I was genuinely pleased. She did, however, offer one suggestion: to try Portobello mushrooms. I thought that idea outrageous at the time—and wasn't my soup already delicious?" But since change can be fun, I decided to give it a try. I hope you will, too.

Portobello Mushroom Barley Soup with Beef

Makes 3 1/2 quarts

1 1/2 pounds beef shank bone with a good amount of meat and marrow*
1 scant cup dried great northern beans or cannellini* - rinsed
1/2 cup uncooked barley - rinsed
1 large onion, diced
4 to 5 carrots, diced
2 large stocks celery, diced
8 ounces Portobello mushroom caps cut into ¼-inch pieces
1/3 cup diced parsley - flat leaf variety preferred
1/4 teaspoon salt
1/4 to 1/2 teaspoon black pepper
2 Tablespoons chicken bouillon base of good quality
2 1/2 quarts water

Trim meat of surrounding fat. Place bone with meat and marrow in a 5 or 6 quart soup pot. Add water. Cover pot and bring to a boil.

Skim top of broth. With lid off, on medium heat, allow broth to reduce a little to concentrate flavor, about 30 minutes.

Add beans and barley. Cover pot and simmer 1 1/2 hour.

Remove meat and bone from pot, discarding the connective tissue. Cut meat in little chunks. Remove marrow from bone and mash with a fork. Discard bone. Return meat and marrow to pot. Continue simmering until meat and beans are almost tender.

Add onion, carrots, celery, mushrooms, soup base, and seasonings; continue simmering about 30 or 40 minutes until meat and mushrooms are nice and tender.

Taste and correct seasonings by adding more of the bullion base, salt, or pepper if needed. (Soup is not meant to be spicy.) Add parsley, and simmer five minutes longer to meld flavors.

When finished, soup should coat a spoon. To thicken, simply remove lid and simmer a little longer. Soup will also thicken overnight.

*If cholesterol is a concern, you may want to discard the marrow along with the bones. Soup will still retain good bit of flavor.

*It is best to soak cannellini beans overnight to shorten cooking time.

Chef's Tips: Onion, carrots and celery can be diced together in a food processor.

Bullion base + tasting are key here. My favorite brand is Better Than Bullion Reduced Sodium Chicken Base.

Not too long ago, I used to make a really serious Italian-style meat sauce, which I would serve over traditional spaghetti-style pasta—accompanied with grated parmesan cheese, hunks of French bread, and a simple green salad. Sounds good? It was! But due to the influx of my children's generation, who are turning into vegans or eating no red meat, I tweaked the recipe and substituted meat with vegetables. The result—no modesty here—was really quite amazing. Not only is it delicious, but also so darn guiltless and nutritious that you could serve it to the surgeon general, who would probably applaud and ask you for a printout.

I hope you will try it. You will never miss the meat. But don't forget the grated cheese for those who might indulge—it tastes great with it. A glass of red wine is not bad either.

Incredible Veggie Pasta Sauce

Makes 1 1/2 quarts

6 ounces Cremini mushrooms, (baby bellas) coarsely diced
1 medium zucchini - coarsely diced
9 ounces frozen artichoke hearts - coarsely diced

The above ingredients together should yield approximately 1 pound, 5 ounces.

1 large celery stock - diced
1/2 large bell pepper - about 3/4 cup, diced
2 1/2 cups diced onion
9 or 10 large cloves garlic diced (no kidding here)
1/2 cup extra virgin olive oil
1 14.5 ounce can diced tomatoes - do not drain
1 8 ounce can tomato sauce
1 6 ounce can tomato paste
1 Tablespoon crushed dried basil
1 Tablespoon crushed dried oregano
1/4 teaspoon salt
1/8 teaspoon black pepper (this is not meant to be spicy)

In Dutch oven, sauté celery, bell pepper, onion and garlic in olive oil for just a few minutes.

Add mushrooms, zucchini, artichokes, salt and pepper. Stir and sauté a few minutes longer.

Add all the tomato ingredients; simmer 10 minutes.

Add dried herbs. Continue simmering 5 minutes longer—stirring a few times just to meld flavors. Taste and correct seasonings.

Allow sauce to sit on warm for 5 minutes. Sauce will thicken nicely. Serve over your favorite pasta, preferably whole wheat.

A green salad is the perfect accompaniment before or during this meal. And don't forget to pass the Parmesan cheese!

Chef's Tips: Dried herbs, such as oregano and basil, release more of their flavor when gently crushed in the palm of your hand before using.

A food processor may be used to dice garlic, onion, celery, zucchini and mushrooms. Artichokes and bell peppers should be cut with a knife.

.

This is not architecture. Veggies do not have to be even or perfectly diced. Relax and enjoy your cooking!

"Bircher Muesli" traces its origin to Switzerland. It was invented by a Dr. Bircher-Benner around 1900 for patients at his world famous clinic in Zurich. He was a true pioneer in the belief that health care went beyond just medicine. I first discovered it at a family owned deli about 25 years ago. It was very rich and delicious—almost like a dessert. I desperately wanted to learn how to make it, but the proprietor was not the least bit forthcoming. Sheer determination propelled me into figuring it out (this was long before dry muesli appeared in the grocery stores) and I've been a fan ever since. A few other people I know are, too. My daughter once took a bowl of it camping, and my best friend asked for a week's supply immediately following her back surgery. She likes hers with milk and raisins—nothing more and nothing less. Best of all, my husband (a carnivore at heart) has taken it up for breakfast!

My recipe is a much lighter version of the one I encountered at the deli, but I think it equally delicious. If you like oatmeal, I urge you to try this. It's quick and versatile with just the right nutrients to jump-start your day.

Marilyn's Lite and Luscious Bircher Muesli

Quick cooking rolled oats - whatever amount you like
Vanilla soy milk or 1% milk - enough to well cover the oats
Raisins or any dried fruit of your choice - small amount
Pecan or walnut pieces - small amount
Agave Nectar* or other sweetener of choice - optional

*Agave Nectar is a product that comes from the Agave plant in Mexico—the same plant that produces tequila. Its main pollinator is the lesser long-nosed bat. It has a low glycemic index, is simple to use, and does not change the taste of anything.

Put rolled oats in a refrigerator container. Pour milk or soymilk over the oats until covered. Add dried fruit, nuts, and sweetener of choice—if using. Stir well to incorporate all of the ingredients. Cover with lid; refrigerate overnight. Stir before serving.

Serve cold.

Mixture will keep several days in the refrigerator.

Chef's Tip: Take advantage of seasonal fresh fruit. I often make up a large batch with just the milk or soy milk, and the oats. The next day I can add whatever I want. A bowl topped with a variety of fresh fruit and a sprinkling of nuts is a great little summertime breakfast or lunch.

Equally delicious and nutritious is frozen fruit. Try it semi-frozen; tastes like ice cream.

About 10 years ago I stunned my family by telling them I would no longer be making the party green bean casserole for dinner. I knew this would not go over well, but I stood my ground. I had excitedly been working on a lovely pea and mushroom dish to replace it. On Thanksgiving, a few cousins strode into the house with picket signs in protest. I was supposed to see the humor in that. I didn't. At the table a cousin-in-law remarked that "…peas are not eaten on Thanksgiving." As if that wasn't enough, a new young family member informed me that "…at Thanksgiving, sweet potatoes should always have marshmallows on the top." At that point I decided to have another glass of wine. But then I noticed my little grandson in his high chair, having just mastered the technique of eating with a spoon, could not get those peas down fast enough. Suddenly, nothing else mattered. I got up from the table and gave my grandson a hug.

The following year I came out with my new and healthy green bean recipe. It was a keeper. As for the young family member, I created a sweet potato dish just for him. I named it Scott's Sweet Potatoes. It has marshmallows on the top.

Thanksgiving Green Beans

Serves 12

2 pounds green beans - whole, stem ends removed
2 cups reduced-sodium chicken broth
6 cloves garlic, diced
2 Tablespoons olive oil
Dash black pepper
Dash salt

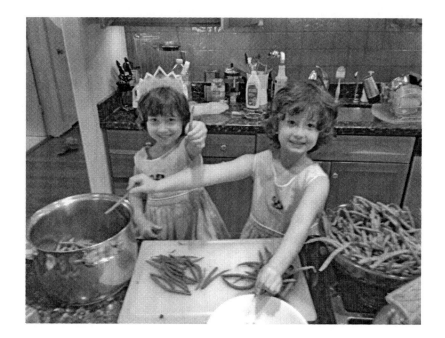

In Dutch oven, or large skillet with lid, sauté garlic in olive oil—just a minute or two. Add chicken broth, green beans, and seasonings. Bring to a boil. Stir. Cover pot with lid and simmer 15 to 20 minutes, or until green beans are al dente (done), but not soft. Taste and correct seasonings if necessary. Stir again and allow green beans to sit covered on warm heat until serving time.

I make these green beans all year. For Thanksgiving, because of the abundance of food that is served, I usually figure that one pound of green beans will serve 6.

Chef's Tips: The secret to this simple recipe is fresh green beans.

For large quantities, baste green beans just before serving with a turkey baster. Discard remaining liquid and serve.

Eating fish is a great way to get protein without the higher concentration of saturated fat found in many cuts of meat. Cold water fatty fish, such as salmon, mackerel, and sardines, are also excellent sources of omega 3 fatty acids we have heard so much about. Besides the claims of being good for the heart, they have also been linked to eye and brain health. Fortunately, salmon seems to be more available these days in both the wild and farm-raised varieties. Because of its diet (it eats directly from the food chain), the wild variety usually has a high concentration of these fats. It is also more expensive. I eat both, depending on the source, the price, and the way it looks. If in doubt it is perfectly acceptable to ask if you can smell the fish, and oftentimes I do.

Since I like the combination of salmon and spinach (Popeye can you hear me?), I came up with this recipe. This spinach pesto (the topping) is a much lighter version of the real thing, because I have omitted the traditional pine nuts and parmesan cheese by substituting bread crumbs and fennel—a very nutritious and savory herb with a subtle licorice flavor. You will never miss the extra calories!

This is a lovely way to serve salmon and particularly nice for company, since the entire dish can be prepared the day before. You can even cook it on a grill, with or without a lid. Either way, the end result is beautiful and delicious.

Sensational Salmon with Spinach Pesto

Serves 6 to 7

Approximately 1 1/2 pounds salmon filet - skin removed.

Marinade:

Approximately 1 1/2 Tablespoons of lemon or lime juice
A couple dashes of reduced sodium soy sauce
A couple dashes of Worcestershire sauce
A couple dashes of cayenne pepper or hot sauce

Mix above ingredients in a small bowl. Pour over salmon and set aside while you prepare the pesto.

Spinach Pesto:

5 ounces fresh spinach leaves - torn in small pieces
2 to 3 small garlic cloves - peeled and quartered
Handful of fennel bulb - about 2 ounces, cut in small pieces
1/8 cup bread crumbs
2 Tablespoons extra virgin olive oil
1/4 teaspoon salt - a few dashes of black pepper

Place all of the above ingredients in a food processor or blender; process until a smooth paste is formed. Taste and correct seasonings.

Preheat oven to 375 degrees.

Lightly coat a long piece of aluminum foil with cooking spray. Place foil over a cookie sheet with oiled side up. Lift salmon from marinade and center on foil. Cover entire filet with pesto until you have a layer about 1/8-inch thick. The remaining pesto can be frozen and used for a smaller filet.

Completely cover salmon with a second piece of foil, keeping all sides open to vent. Bake 18 to 20 minutes. Remove from oven and allow salmon to sit a few minutes before serving.

Equally delicious hot or cold.

Chef's Tip: Pesto can be frozen. The entire recipe can be prepared the day before and refrigerated. On the day of serving, bring to room temperature. Bake in preheated oven.

Use the rest of the fennel bulb in spinach salads. It pairs well with orange.

While chicken breasts are an excellent choice of low-fat meat, they sometimes taste a little dry—often the result of overcooking. You do not want to undercook the meat either, causing toughness. It is important to slice across the grain. Slicing across the grain shortens the fibers and provides a more tender, succulent piece of meat.

In this recipe, the chicken breast is kissed with just the right amount of lemon juice and wine—delivering extra moisture and flavor to the meat. It is further enhanced by the richness of the extra virgin olive oil and luscious Shiitake mushrooms. This is my most recent chicken recipe using only white meat—one I expect to be making often. I believe you will like it, too.

Glazed Chicken Breasts with Shiitake Mushrooms

Serves 4

1 pound skinless, boneless chicken breasts cut into 4 large pieces
6 ounces shiitake mushrooms, sliced or quartered
1/4 cup diced onion
3 cloves garlic - diced
1/4 cup extra virgin olive oil
1/3 cup white wine, such as chardonnay
2 Tablespoons fresh lemon juice
Lowry salt, or seasoning of choice
Black pepper

Lightly season chicken on both sides with Lawry salt and black pepper.

In large skillet, allow oil to come to temperature. Over medium heat, sauté chicken on both sides until lightly browned. Remove from skillet and set aside.

Stir fry garlic, onion and mushrooms in remaining oil for a few minutes. Season lightly.

Turn heat to low and slowly pour in wine. Return chicken to pan. Pour lemon juice over chicken and mushrooms. Cover pan with lid and simmer over medium low heat 8 minutes. Turn chicken and give mushrooms a good stir. Continue simmering another 8 minutes or until chicken is tender.

Turn off heat and stir in parsley.
Plate chicken and drizzle mushrooms and any remaining juices over chicken. Excellent with brown rice and Thanksgiving Green Beans - page 100.

Chef's Tips: Shiitake mushrooms are very flavorful and offer a lot of nice rich texture to this dish. The dried ones are much more affordable and convenient. You can find them in the Asian section of most supermarkets. Just be sure to remove all stems on shiitakes and follow directions on package for reconstituting. You can freeze what you don't use. They are delicious in omelets.

There seems to be even more evidence today of the role plants play in keeping our bodies healthy. One of the techniques I employ to add a variety of colorful vegetables to my diet is cooking three or four together in one pot. Not only does it look appealing, it also reduces clean-up time. When you are in the grocery store shopping, think color, and don't be afraid to experiment. That is how this recipe came about.

Tri-Colored Chayote Squash

Serves 4

2 good-size Chayote squash - about 1.5 pounds total
1 large red bell pepper - stems and seeds removed
1 large orange bell pepper - stem and seeds removed
4 cloves diced garlic
3 or 4 scallions - green part only, cut in thirds
2 Tablespoons extra virgin olive oil
Salt and black pepper to taste.
A good pinch of dried tarragon - optional

Cut squash in half lengthwise and remove seeds. Slice squash and bell peppers lengthwise into nice long strips—about ½-inch wide.

In a large skillet, warm oil over medium low heat. Add squash. Season lightly with salt, black pepper, and tarragon. Turn heat to low and sauté squash about 5 minutes, turning one time. Stir in bell peppers and garlic. Lightly season again with salt and pepper. Cover with lid and continue cooking until all vegetables are al dente (done, but not limp.) Stir in scallions and serve immediately.

Chef's Tip: Bell peppers should be firm at time of purchase.

I adore mango! Consequently, I am always pondering different ways to use this succulent fruit—a gift to us from the tropics.

Therefore, on one of those great days when everything seemed to be working right, I came up with this extraordinary combination for a stir-fry dinner. It was perfect on my first attempt. I thought to myself, *Am I getting better at this, or is this just a stroke of luck?*

Admittedly, this recipe does take some time, but I think the result is well worth it. You will love the way the exotic flavors of ginger, mango and cilantro come together with the broccoli, carrots and beef. And because it looks so pretty in the skillet, I always have my guests plate it themselves.

A good way to save time and work for yourself when preparing meals such as this is to partner with a family member. My husband usually dices the onion, garlic, ginger and cilantro whenever I am fixing this dish. My son and daughter-in-law often cook together too, and seem to enjoy it. My daughter engages her 14-year-old son as her sous chef. Her husband prefers to do the cleanup, claiming it's therapeutic. I'll vote for that!

Outrageous Beef and Mango Stir-fry

Serves 4 to 5

3/4 pound flank steak, top sirloin, or other tender cut of beef
2 Tablespoons peanut oil
1/2 cup chicken broth

2 1/4 cups carrots, cut in ½-inch pieces
2 1/2 cups broccoli florets
1/3 cup diced onion
1/2 Tablespoons diced ginger
4 large cloves of diced garlic

1 Tablespoon cornstarch
1/2 cup chicken broth
1 Tablespoon sherry
1 to 2 Tablespoons reduced sodium soy sauce
1 or 2 dashes of cayenne pepper
1 teaspoon fresh lemon juice

1 large ripe but firm mango, cut in small chunks
1/3 cup diced cilantro

Slice flank steak thin and <u>on the diagonal</u>. Cut in 2-inch strips.

In your largest skillet or sauté pan, heat oil over medium high heat until smoking point.

Brown steak quickly on each side. Remove and set aside.

Deglaze skillet by adding 1/2 cup chicken broth and simmering a few minutes.

Add carrots, broccoli, onion, ginger and garlic to pan. Cover with lid, and cook over medium heat until vegetables are crisp tender—about 8 minutes.

Meantime, dissolve cornstarch in remaining chicken broth. Stir in sherry, soy, cayenne pepper, and lemon juice. Add to pan and stir well. Mixture will thicken a little.

Return beef to skillet, stir, and simmer over low heat a couple minutes. Stir in mango, followed by cilantro. Serve hot over rice.

Chef's Tips: Have beef and mango at room temperature.

When mangos come into season, I love to find different ways to use them. And, I openly confess to hanging over the sink gnawing on that sweet and succulent part you simply can't get off. It must be a primal instinct left over from one of my ancestors.

This mango creation is turning out to be one of my favorite side dishes. It seems to go well with everything, and it has zero fat. The first time I served it was at a small dinner party for friends, along with a light shrimp and hearts of palm salad. It got raves! For an appetizer, we had guacamole.

One of the many attributes about mangos is that they aide in digestion, making them a happy pairing with black beans—plus, a superb twosome for maintaining good blood sugar levels.

But try this salad just for the taste of it. You will find the tart and sweet contrast interesting and delicious. And since it is easy to fix and looks so pretty, you will want to take it to your next pot luck. I am!

Black Bean and Mango Salad

Serves 6

2 16 ounce cans black beans
1/3 cup diced onion
1/2 cup diced red bell pepper
1 small jalapeno pepper seeded and diced
1/2 cup diced cilantro or fresh basil
3 Tablespoons lime juice
1/2 teaspoon seasoned rice vinegar
1/4 teaspoon salt
1 large ripe but firm mango cut in small cubes

Thoroughly rinse beans in cold water—drain well. Place all ingredients, in order given, into a large salad bowl. Toss together with a plastic spatula or wooden spoon, being careful not to mash beans or mango in the process.

Refrigerate a few hours, or overnight, to thicken a little and meld flavors. Serve with a slotted spoon.

Chef's Tip: A simple way to blend delicate ingredients together is by tossing back and forth into another large bowl, stirring in between. This is especially helpful when preparing large batches of potato salad, or just about anything.

This lovely vegetable combination arrived on our dinner plates the evening of my son's birthday. I wanted something green and crunchy to go with the tender osso buco (veal shanks) and pasta dish I was planning. It was perfect.

Sugar snap peas and snow peas are both in the legume family, and that means plenty of vitamins, minerals and fiber for you. The next time you want to add a little texture to your meal, try this delicious combo. By preparing the vegetables and almonds ahead of time, it's sure to be a snap.

Sugar Snap Pea, Snow Pea, and Green Bean Sauté

Serves 6 to 7

1/3 cup almond slivers
1/2 pound of fresh sugar snap peas
2 1/2 Tablespoons walnut oil
1/2 pound of fresh snow peas
1/2 pound of fresh green beans
1/4 teaspoon dried thyme or equivalent of fresh if you have it
1/4 teaspoon salt

*Walnut oil intensifies the flavor of this lovely dish, but you can certainly substitute olive oil and it will still be delicious.

Preheat oven to 400. Spread almonds evenly on foil or pan. Place in oven on middle rack and toast about three minutes. Pay attention, as they burn quickly. Set aside to cool. Store in a plastic bag until using.

Remove stem ends from green beans. Blanch green beans and sugar snap peas together by immersing in a large pot of boiling water for two minutes. Immediately add snow peas and continue cooking for one minute. Drain and plunge in ice water a few seconds to stop the cooking process. Drain and pat the vegetables dry with a cloth or paper towel. Place in a plastic bag and set aside or refrigerate.

Bring veggies to room temperature.

Heat oil in a large skillet or sauté pan over medium heat. Stir in green beans and peas. Sprinkle with the thyme and salt, and continue stirring until green beans and peas are heated. Sprinkle with toasted almonds and serve.

Herbs 101: Always crush dried herbs in the palm of your hand before adding to any dish; this will release their full flavor.

Chef's Tip: Neither sugar snap peas or snow peas need any preparation or shelling.

Tilapia Taco Party

This identical party took place at my son's house one evening. While I was busy getting everything ready, guests helped themselves to guacamole and chips. The recipe for the guacamole came from a friend. She said the extra little pop comes from the Worcestershire sauce. Who would have known?

Most people love guacamole—even young children, if not too spicy. And now you can find low-fat, low-sodium chips at most supermarkets.

Go for it! Have a taco party.

Awesome Guacamole

Serves 16

8 ripe but firm large avocados
8 to 10 cherry tomatoes finely diced - seeds okay
1/2 cup freshly squeezed lemon or lime juice
Approx. 1/8 cup finely diced onion
1 or 2 cloves minced garlic
Dash black pepper
1/4 teaspoon Worcestershire sauce
A few good dashes hot sauce
1/2 teaspoon salt

With peel on, halve avocados lengthwise. Twist and remove pit. With a large spoon, scoop out fruit in one big piece. Coarsely mash avocados with a fork until desired consistency.

Add remaining ingredients; blend all together. Taste to correct seasonings and juice, if needed. Refrigerate until serving time.

Chef's Tips: A food processor works very well for large amounts. Strive for a little texture; most people like guacamole chunky.

A little lemon or lime juice on top will keep it from turning dark. Simply stir at serving.

Tilapia Tacos

Makes 12 to16 tacos

Preheat oven to 375 degrees.

Brush 4 or 5 nice tilapia filets (or other mild fish) on each side with olive oil. Lightly season each side with salt, garlic granules, and cayenne pepper. Place fish on a cookie sheet lined with foil. Turn up ends and sides of foil to catch any drippings.

Bake fish 15 minutes. Remove from oven and add a bit more olive oil if fish seems a little dry. Dribble each filet with freshly squeezed lime juice. Divide each filet into 3 or 4 portions. Place on platter with serving utensil.

Ingredients for each fish taco:

Arugula or lettuce - cut up*
Cherry or plum tomatoes - cut in very small pieces and lightly salted
Diced scallions or red onions
Cilantro
Jalapeno - seeded and diced
Avocado - diced (optional); a little lemon juice keeps it from turning dark

While fish is baking, place each of the above ingredients in six individual small bowls, along with six small serving spoons. Place toppings beside fish for guests to help themselves.

Tortillas: Quickly warm 12 to 16 tortillas (depending on the size) and bring to the buffet. You can do this in a microwave—takes only a few seconds—by stacking in a small covered dish or wrapped in a paper napkin.

Have a salt shaker handy and a bottle of hot sauce, for those who like it.

*Equally delicious with just plain store-bought coleslaw.

Chef's Tips: When shopping, be sure to buy plenty of toppings so you don't run out; leftover toppings are delicious over tuna, chicken or cheese.

If possible, order tortillas from Mexican restaurants or local panderias (Mexican bakeries) that don't use preservatives. They are less expensive and usually taste better. You can freeze the ones you don't use. Children love them with scrambled eggs.

For dessert I highly recommend the "Banana Dark Chocolate with Toasted Walnuts Muffin," on page 116.

This recipe was challenging; I knew what I was after, yet time and time again I would find a little flaw. I began comparing myself to Thomas Edison and his 1,000 unsuccessful attempts to create a light bulb. Without my husband's encouragement to carry on (he got to eat the rejects), I'm sure I would not be offering this little melt-in-your-mouth, delicious treat today. Like my very popular, "One's a Meal Muffin" on page 84, I use no preservatives, only whole grains, very little cholesterol, and mostly healthy fats. The agave nectar—a processed form of natural sugar, has a low glycemic index. This means it is slowly absorbed into the body, preventing blood sugar spikes. And because agave nectar is about 1 1/2 times sweeter than regular sugar, you can use less. Another plus—agave does not change the taste of anything, the reason children like it.

As in the "One's a Meal Muffins," this recipe uses the standard 12-cup muffin pan. Because of young grandchildren, I bake mine in a little smaller size cup using two pans. This yields 18 nice little muffins. I simply fill the remaining cups with about an inch of water to keep from burning the pan. The baking temperature for this size remains the same; the time (depending on your oven) is about 25 to 26 minutes, or until tested clean.

Banana Dark Chocolate Muffins with Toasted Walnuts

Yields 12 to 18 muffins

1 cup very ripe bananas or 10 ounces
1 cup vanilla soy milk
1/4 cup canola oil
1 large egg*
2/3 cup minus 1/2 teaspoon organic agave nectar
1/4 teaspoon vanilla

1cup whole wheat pastry flour*
1 teaspoon baking soda
1/2 teaspoon salt
1cup quick cooking rolled oats
1/2 cup minus 2 teaspoons wheat bran
1/2 cup minus 2 teaspoons oat bran
1/2 cup toasted walnut pieces*
1/3 to1/2 cup dark chocolate chips

Preheat oven to 325 degrees.

Puree bananas in a blender or food processor. Add vanilla soy, oil, egg, agave nectar, and vanilla. Process until blended and smooth.

In large mixing bowl, mix together pastry flour, baking soda, and salt. Stir in rest of the dry ingredients, blending all together.

Add wet ingredients to the dry. Follow with the nuts and chocolate chips. With a wooden spoon mix all ingredients together until no trace of flour remains. **Do not beat.** Allow to set a few minutes before filling pans.

Pour mixture into a lightly oiled muffin pan that yields 12. Bake about 26 minutes or until tested clean. Remove pan from oven and place on a rack to cool, about 15 minutes.

Remove muffins from pan by gently loosening sides with a dinner knife. Muffins will slide out nicely. Place on rack until completely cooled. Freeze extras for family and friends in ziplock bag.

*Eggs 101: If you are concerned about cholesterol, use 1 large omega 3 fortified egg, or 1/4 cup egg substitute, or 2 large egg whites.

*Toasted walnuts: Preheat oven to 400 degrees. Spread walnuts on a medium-size pan covered with foil. Bake nuts until lightly browned, about 3 to 4 minutes. Remove from oven and set aside to cool.

*Pastry flour imparts a more delicate texture to breads and muffins.

Chef's Tip: Extra scrumptious when warmed in microwave.

Notes

2, 63   *Vital to the emotional and physical health of our youth*
Richard Louv, *Last Child in the Woods,* "Nature Deficit Disorder and the Restorative Environment," (Chapel Hill, NC: Algonquin Books, 2008) 99-112.

Chapter 1 – What You Need to Know

6   *What are Discretionary Calories?*
United States Department of Agriculture, "Inside the Pyramid: adapted from What are Discretionary Calories?" MyPyramid Food Guidance System, October 8, 2008,
http://www.mypyramid.gov/pyramid/discretionary_calories.html.

7   *Why is physical activity important?*
United States Department of Agriculture, Physical Activity: adapted from "Why is physical activity important?" http://www.choosemyplate.gov/physical-activity/why.html, (accessed November 9, 2012).

8   *"There are four types of pineapples"*
United States Department of Health and Human Services Centers for Disease Control and Prevention, "Fruit of the Month: Pineapple," Varieties,
http://www.fruitsandveggiesmatter.gov/month/pineapple.html.

8   *Save wintering songbirds*
Bridget Stutchbury, "Put A Songbird on Your Shopping List," *National Wildlife Magazine* 47, no. 1 (Dec/ Jan 2009), Also available online at
http://www.nwf.org/NationalWildlife/article.cfm?issueID=126&articleID=1668.

Chapter 2 – Tips and Techniques

Tips for Making Great Shakes

11   *"Red blush on fruit depends on the variety"*
North Carolina Department of Agriculture & Consumer Services, "Peaches," Horticultural Crops, October 8, 2008, http://www.ncagr.gov/markets/commodit/horticul/peaches/.

12   *"Maintain high quality for 8 to 12 months."*
William Schafer and Shirley T. Munson, "Freezing Fruits and Vegetables: Storage Times for Frozen Fruits and Vegetables," Reviewed 2009, University Of Minnesota Extension,
http://www1.extension.umn.edu/food-safety/preserving/fruits/freezing-fruit.

Chapter 4 – Make a Shake

The Black Bear

26   *dined on blueberries and venison*
Jane Ammeson, "Pick Health, Pick Blueberries," *The Northwest Indiana and Illinois Times Newspaper,* July 6, 2005, http://www.nwitimes.com/articles/2005/07/06/
features/food/2cf94b47d0af51d486257032001cd72d.prt.

26   *The secret lies in its deep, purple-blue color*
U.S. Highbush Blueberry Council, "Health Benefits of Blueberries," Blueberry Nutrition Research, Blueberries contain substances that have antioxidant properties,
http://www.blueberrycouncil.com/health-benefits-of-blueberries/blueberry-nutrition/,
(accessed July 1, 2013).

First Class Hibernator

27   *In the fall, fruit, nuts, and acorns*
Tanya Dewey and Christine Kronk, "Ursus Americanus," Food Habits, Animal Diversity Web, 2007,
http://animaldiversity.ummz.umich.edu/site/accounts/information/Ursus_americanus.html.

27   *"Female bears give birth during hibernation"*
Mark D. Jones, "What's in a Name? Hibernation Means Different Things to Different Animals," North Carolina
Wildlife Resources Commission, April 1999.
http://216.27.39.101/Wildlife_Species_Con/WSC_Black_Bear_hibernate.htm.

The Bat

28   *More mangos are eaten fresh around the world*
Sam Gugino, "All About Mangos," Sam on Fruit, http://www.samcooks.com/food/
fruit/mangoes.html.

28   *Cultivated in India about 4000 years ago*
Natural History Museum London, "Mango: Origins of Cultivation," Nature Online: Seeds of Trade, 2007,
www.nhm.ac.uk/jdsml/nature-online/seeds-of-
trade/page.dsml?section=regions&ref=mango.

28   *An excellent source of antioxidants*
United States Department of Health and Human Services Centers for Disease Control and Prevention, "Fruit of
the Month: Mango," Fruits and Veggies Matter,
http://www.fruitsandveggiesmatter.gov/month/mango.html.

Nature s Number 1 Pest Controller

29   *"Bats very rarely carry rabies."*
Diana Fosse (Texas Parks and Wildlife), e-mail message to author, April 2009.

29   *"Can eat more than 1,000 mosquito-sized insects;" that a lot of our favorite fruits; called "farmers of the tropics"*
Bat Conservation International, "Benefits of Bats: Pest Control, Pollinators, Seed Dispersers," Updated April1,
2011, http://www.batcon.org/index.php/all-about-bats/intro-
to-bats/subcategory/18.html.

The Bee

30   *Just eight medium size berries*
Denise Mann, "Health and Nutrition Information," *Los Angeles Daily News: L.A. Life*, July 14, 1997, Also available
online at http://www.berrypatchfarm.com/health.htm.

30   *200 seeds in a strawberry*
University of Illinois Extension, "Strawberries and More: Facts," Urban Programs Resource Network,
http://www.urbanext.uiuc.edu/strawberries/facts.cfm.

The Pollinator

31   *The purpose of a flower; it must have help*
Adapted from Nature 101: Wildflowers and Pollination, Houston Arboretum & Nature
Center, Houston, TX. 1996.

31   *Many flowers also have U V patterns*
Cynthia Berger, "What Are Bugs Worth?" Nature Watch: A Bee's-Eye View, *National Wildlife Magazine* 44, no. 6 (Oct/Nov 2006), Also available online at http://www.nwf.org/News-and-Magazines/National-Wildlife/Animals/Archives/2006/What-Are-Bugs-Worth.aspx.

31   *Other important thing*
Pat Marks, "Pollination" (5th grade curriculum, Houston Arboretum & Nature Center, Houston, TX. 2003).

31   *No native North American honeybees*
Charles C. Mann, "America Found & Lost," *National Geographic,* May 2007,
Also available on line at
http://www.charlesmann.org/articles/NatGeo-Jamestown-05-07-2.htm.

The Hummingbird

32   *Story begins with Christopher Columbus; also a sign of welcome and friendship*
Julia F. Morton, Miami, FL. "Pineapple, Ananas comosus;" Origin and Distribution, p. 18–28, In: Fruits of Warm Climates, 1987; Horticulture and Landscape Architecture, Purdue University: Center for New Crops and Plant Products, http://www.hort.purdue.edu/newcrop/morton/pineapple.html.

32   *Refrigeration on ships was non-existent; "that made the trip home were very prized;" "was truly an honor"*
Guest Services, Inc., "The Pineapple: A Symbol of Hospitality,"
http://www.guestservices.com/logo-pineapple.

32   *A gesture of great cordiality*
Hoag Levins, "Social History of the Pineapple: Pineapple as Hospitality Symbol,"
http://www.levins.com/pineapple.html.

32   *Other reasons for placing the pineapple on a pedestal*
American Academy of Anti-Aging Medicine, "Bromelain (Pineapple Enzyme)," Anti-Aging Desk Reference: Other Vital Nutraceuticals & Nutrients, posted December 31,2005,
http://www.worldhealth.net/news/bromelain_pineapple_enzyme.

32   *An excellent source of vitamin C*
United States Department of Health and Human Services Centers for Disease Control and Prevention, "Fruit of the Month: Pineapple," Fruits and Veggies Matter,
http://www.fruitsandveggiesmatter.gov/month/pineapple.html.

The Little Helicopter

33   *Very important pollinators of wildflowers*
United States Forest Service, "Celebrating Wildflowers: Bird Pollination,"
http://www.fs.fed.us/wildflowers/pollinators/animals/birds.shtml.

33   *A bird bath with a few small rocks*
Doreen Cubie, "Creating a Haven for Hummingbirds," *National Wildlife Magazine* 40, no. 6 (Oct/Nov 2002). Also available online at http://www.nwf.org/News-and-Magazines/National-Wildlife/Gardening/Archives/2002/Creating-a-Haven-for-Hummingbirds.aspx.

33   *"About 10 feet from dense shrubs or other cover"*
National Wildlife Federation, "Garden For Wildlife: Making Wildlife Habitat At Home,"
Create a Bird-friendly Habitat, http://www.nwf.org/Get-Outside/Outdoor-Activities/Garden-for-Wildlife/Gardening-Tips/How-to-Attract-Birds-to-Your-Garden.aspx.

The Orangutan

34   *"One of the earliest fruits"*
Mary King, "Florida Food Fare," Family & Consumer Sciences, University of Florida/ IFAS, Sarasota County Extension, http://sarasota.extension.ufl.edu/fcs/FlaFoodFare/Figs.pdf (accessed July 16, 2010).

34   *"Have been around for at least 6,000 years"*
Mary King, "Florida Food Fare," Family & Consumer Sciences, University of Florida/ IFAS, Sarasota County Extension, http://sarasota.extension.ufl.edu/fcs/FlaFoodFare/Figs.pdf
(accessed July 16, 2010).

Man of the Forest

35   *"Highly intelligent" animals that can solve problems; "share 96.4% of our DNA"*
Man of the Forest (Helen Buckland), "About Orangutans: Man of the Forest,"
http://www.manoftheforest.com/Manoftheforest/aboutorangutans.

35   *Craft their own tools*
Jennifer Horton, how stuff works, A Discovery Company, "Are orangutans introverts?,"
"Tricks of the Trade And Disappearing Act," (Cawthon Lang, K/June 13, 2005), available on line at
http://animals.howstuffworks.com/mammals/orangutan-introversion.htm/printable, (accessed June 20, 2011).

35   *Know where to find their favorite fruit*
St. Louis Zoo, "Sumatran Orangutan: A Passion for Fruit,"
http://www.stlzoo.org/animals/abouttheanimals/mammals/lemursmonkeysapes/sumatranorangutan.htm.

35   *Are "critically endangered"*
The Nature Conservancy, Hawaii, "Pacific Connections: Hanging with the Orangutans,"
http://www.nature.org/ourinitiatives/regions/northamerica/unitedstates/hawaii/explore/the-nature-conservancy-in-hawaii-hanging-with-the-orangutans.xml (posted March 01,2011),
also see, Orangutan Crisis - Sumantran Orangutan Society, "The Conservation Status of the Sumantran Orangutan," on line at http://www.orangutans-sos.org/orangutans/crisis/.

35   *Their habitat is rich in biodiversity; ranked as one of the richest in the world*
World Wildlife Fund, Full Report, (2011) "Sumatran lowland rainforests (IM0158)," online at
http://www.worldwildlife.org/wildworld/profiles/terrestrial/im/im0158_full.html,
also see World Wildlife Fund, Full Report, (2011) "Borneo lowland rain forests (IM0102)," on line at
http://www.worldwildlife.org/wildworld/profiles/terrestrial/im/im0102_full.html.
Both reports originally published in the book: Terrestrial Eco regions of the Indo-Pacific: a conservation assessment from Island Press.

35   *"Gardeners of the forest;" "crucial role in forest regeneration"*
Sumatran Orangutan Society, "About Orangutans: Orangutan Crisis," Threats, Illegal Trade,
(posted 2008), http://www.orangutans-sos.org/orangutans/crisis/.

35   *Leaders of three nations that share Borneo*
World Wildlife Fund, "Nations Sign Historic Declaration to Save   Heart of Borneo ," *Focus* 29, no. 3 (May/ June 2007), 1, Also available online at
www.worldwildlife.org/who/focus/WWFBinaryitem7534.pdf.

The Cardinal

36   *Providing 50% of our daily value requirement; medium to bright red, and in unstained cartons*
United States Department of Health and Human Services Centers for Disease Control and Prevention, Fruit and Vegetable of the Month: Berries, "Selection," Fruits and Veggies Matter,
http://www.fruitsandveggiesmatter.gov/month/berries.html.

The Performer

37   *They are monogamous*
Paul Ehrlich, David S. Dobkin and Darryl Wheye, "Northern Cardinal," in The Birders Handbook: A Field Guide to the Natural History of North American Birds (New York: Simon & Schuster Inc., 1988), 554.

37   *This enchanting act is known as the "cardinal kiss"*
Bird Watcher's Digest.com, Bill Thompson, "Top 10 Reasons Spring Feeding is Great: 7. Courtship Behavior," Bird, http://www.birdwatchersdigest.com/site/print.php?id=209.

37   *Cardinals are altricial*
Paul Ehrlich, David S. Dobkin and Darryl Wheye, "Northern Cardinal," in The Birders Handbook: A Field Guide to the Natural History of North American Birds (New York: Simon
& Schuster Inc., 1988), 554-555.

37   *Both parents feed the chicks a diet of insects*
Crane, J. 2001. "Cardinalis cardinalis" (On-line), Animal Diversity Web. Accessed June 12, 2012 at http://animaldiversity.ummz.umich.edu/site/accounts/information/Cardinalis_cardinalis.html.

37   *Even the female sings*
The Cornell Lab of Ornithology, "All About Birds: Bird Guide, Northern Cardinal," Cool Facts; Cornell University, http://www.allaboutbirds.org/guide/Northern_cardinal/lifehistory.

37   *"Valued as destroyers of weed seeds"*
Info please, Encyclopedia: finch, *The Columbia Electronic Encyclopedia*, 6th ed., 2007, Columbia University Press, http://www.infoplease.com/ce6/sci/A0818687.html.

The Chickadee

38   *"Contains 90.5% of the daily value for vitamin E."*
Naturally-Healthy-Eating.com [Mary Jane Moses], "Sunflower Seeds Are Packed with Benefits," The Amazing Seed: A Bonanza of Nutritional Benefits
http://www.naturally-healthy-eating.com/sunflower-seeds.html.

The Acrobat

39   *They often hang upside down while feeding on their prey*
Paul Ehrlich, David S. Dobkin and Darryl Wheye, "Songbird," in The Birders Handbook: A Field Guide to the Natural History of North American Birds (New York: Simon & Schuster, Inc., 1988), 381.

39   *Favor the black oil variety of sunflower seed*
The Wild Bird Feeding Industry, "6 Steps to Turn Your Yard into a Sanctuary for Birds,"
Choosing Bird Food: Seed Types http://www.backyardbirdcare.org/step2.html.

39   *Seeds can become rancid*
Naturally-Healthy-Eating.com [Mary Jane Moses], "Sunflower Seeds Are Packed with Benefits: Eating and Storing", http://www.naturally-healthy-eating.com/sunflower- seeds.html.

39   *One of the most sophisticated and varied call system*
Carina Stranton, "Tracking the Vocabulary of Songbirds," July 5, 2005, Also available online at http://seattletimes.nwsource.com/html/localnews/2002357574_chickadee05m.html.

39   *A sizeable dent in the insect population*
Woody Deryckx, "Encouraging Chickadees in the Garden and Orchar4d," *Tilth Producers Quarterly: A Journal of Organic and Sustainable Agriculture*, Spring 1978, Also available online at http://www.tilthproducers.org/tpqpdfs/19.pdf.

The Antelope

40 *Raspberries – an important late summer food source*
Museum <u>Link</u> Illinois, "Mississippian: Economy: Food," Prehistoric / Historic, Illinois State Museum, last updated April 11, 2006, http://www.museum.state.il.us/muslink/nat_amer/pre/htmls/m_food.html.

The Athlete

41 *One of its "best defense strategies against" predators*
Andrea E. Weeks, ed., "Frensley Hall of the Serengetti: Greater Kudo," Houston Museum of Natural Science Guide, 1999,39, ISBN: 0-9640348-1- 6.

41 *It escapes the cheetah, lion, leopard, and other serious enemies*
IMP Publishing Ltd., ed., Wildlife Fact File 1, no. 110 (1994), ISBN: 08-50-04-0016, quoted in Wikipedia The Free Encyclopedia, s.v. "Greater Kudu: Predators," http://en.wikipedia.org/wiki/Greater_Kudu (accessed December 24, 2008).

41 *They also draw in liquid from the plants and fruits they eat*
American Wildlife Foundation, "Kudu: Kudus love to feast on fruits," http://www.awf.org/wildlife-conservation/kudu.

41 *Only the bull (male) grows these graceful spiraling horns*
American Wildlife Foundation, "Kudu: Physical Characteristics," http://www.awf.org/wildlife-conservation/kudu.

The Butterfly

42 *Not only a good source of antioxidants A and C*
North Carolina Department of Agriculture & Consumer Services, "Peaches," Horticultural Crops, October 8, 2008, http://www.ncagr.gov/markets/commodit/horticul/peaches/.

The Transformer

43 *"Butterflies suffer from the same ills that plague all wildlife"*
Heather Millar, "Restoring Rare Beauties," *National Wildlife Magazine* 46, no. 4 (Jun/July 2008), 25. Also available online at
http://www.nwf.org/NationalWildlife/article.cfm?issueID=122&articleID=1596.

43 *When considering food, choose native species*
Houston Arboretum & Nature Center: Nature Center: Special Gardens: Hummingbird and Butterfly Island, http://www.houstonarboretum.org/hummingbirdbutterfly.asp.

43 *"Most butterfly caterpillars are very persnickety eaters"*
Pat Marks [Houston Arboretum & Nature Center], conversation with author, 2003.

The Raccoon

44 *What's in it for you?*
K-State Research and Extension, Family Nutrition Program, *Fruits and Vegetables...Good for You*, Berries!, A Rainbow of Colors, available online at
http://www.ksre.ksu.edu/HumanNutrition/doc9974.ashx.
(accessed June 30, 2013).

On Behalf of the Raccoon

45 *"They eat insects, nuts, worms, frogs,*
Project Wildlife, "Living With Raccoons: Raccoon Facts," http://www.projectwildlife.org/living-raccoons.htm, available on line at roundrocktexas.gov/docs/living_with_raccoons.pdf.

45   *If a raccoon is raiding my garbage can; "capable of traveling great distances"*
Audubon Society of Portland, "Raccoons: Tips on living with Raccoons,"
http://audubonportland.org/wcc/urban/raccoons.

45   *Much better for them; those animals are no longer wild*
Georgia Stigall, "Helping Wildlife...Stay Healthy and Wild," 1996, quoted in Crawdad Creek Wildlife Rehab,
"Feeding Wildlife – Please Don t,"
http://www.geocities.com/crawdadcreekrehab/FeedingWildlife.html.

The Peacock

46   *The deep purple color points to anthocyanins*
North Carolina Department of Agriculture and Consumer Services, "Blackberries," North Carolina Grower/ Shipper Directory,
http://www.agr.state.nc.us/freshconnect/shipperdirectory/blackberry.htm.

The Showoff

47   *"Dry semi-desert grasslands, scrub and deciduous forests; it forages and nests on the ground"*
NYC - Bronx - Bronx Zoo: Blue Peacock, Flickr - Photo Sharing! available on line at
http://www.flickr.com/photos/wallyg/469808373/ (accessed October 15, 2011).

47   *Sometimes, with their chicks on their backs.*
Sheppard Software, "Characteristics & Behavior: Piggy-back Bird," Peafoul,
http://www.sheppardsoftware.com/content/animals/animals/birds/peafowl.htm

47   *Will emit a "screaming alarm cry"*
Rolling Hills Wildlife Adventure, "Common (Indian) Peafowl: Social Structure and Behavior,"
http://www.rollinghillswildlife.com/animals/p/peafowl/.

47   *"Strong short bursts"*
Susan Lumpkin, "At the Zoo: Peafoul," *Smithsonian Zoogoer*, May/June 2000, Also
available online at http://nationalzoo.si.edu/Publications/ZooGoer/2000/3/peafowl.cfm.

47   *"Will eat nearly anything"*
Rolling Hills Wildlife Adventure, "Common (Indian) Peafowl: Diet,"
http://www.rollinghillswildlife.com/animals/p/peafowl/.

47   *A predator to young cobras in domestic communities,*
Rosemary Drisdale, "Facts About Indian Peacocks: Blue Peafoul Feeding Facts," *Suite 101.com*, November 29, 2007,
http://birds.suite101.com/article.cfm/facts_about_indian_peacocks.

47   *"Females are believed to choose their mates"*
National Geographic," Animals, Peacock,
"http://animals.nationalgeographic.com/animals/birds/peacock.html.

47   *"In all sorts of species"*
Matt Ridley, "Modern Darwins: The Father of Evolution would be Thrilled to See the Science His Theory has
Inspired," *National Geographic*, February 2009, Also available online at
http://ngm.nationalgeographic.com/2009/02/darwin-legacy/ridley-text.

Monkey Latte

48   *"Provides more healthful antioxidants"*
Randolf E. Schmid, "Coffee is Good for You After All – In Moderation," *Seattle Times*,
August 30, 2005,
http://seattletimes.nwsource.com/html/nationworld/2002455365_coffee29.html.

The Parrot

50   *Largest producer of pistachios in the world; is California*
Galvin Nussingten, "Enjoyable Truths about Pistachio Nuts," ABC Article Directory,
http://www.abcarticledirectory.com/Article/Enjoyable-Truths-about-Pistachio-Nuts/164588
(accessed August 10, 2012).

The Mimic

51   *"Are at risk of extinction in their native habitats;" Populations of non-native parrots that live in the United States;*
"Only two parrot species"
Jen Uscher, "Finding Refuge in an Urban Jungle," *National Wildlife Magazine* 46, no. 4 (Jun/ Jul 2008): 12-13. Also
available online at http://www.nwf.org/News-and- Magazines/National-Wildlife/Birds/Archives/2008/Parrots-Liv-
ing-Wild-in-American- Cities.aspx.

51   *Not all parrots eat the same thing in the wild; a smorgasbord of seeds, fruit, flowers, nuts, bark*
Race Foster, Marty Smith, and Holly Nash, eds. "Bird Nutrition: Feeding Pet Birds, Parrot Diets, and Nutrition Rec-
ommendations," http://www.peteducation.com/article.cfm?c=15+1835&aid=2844.

51   *"Palm nuts and nuts are their favorites"*
Carolyn Swicegood, The Kitchen Physician, "Nuts Are For the Birds: Vet Recommends Daily Nuts,"
http://www.landofvos.com/articles/NutNutrition.html.

51   *"Their extraordinary beak"; "Only a bird with special adaptations and ingenuity"*
T.J. Lafeber, "Facts & Care; Beaks & Nails: The Incredible Beak," in Let's Celebrate Pet Birds: How to Understand,
Care For and Live Happily with Birds (Odell, IL: Lafeber Co., 1989).Also available online at
http://www.netpets.com/birds/reference/lafeber/8/incredible_beak.html.

51   *Do All Parrots Mimic?*
Michael Schindlinger, "Why do parrots have the ability to mimic?" Scientific American, Ask the Experts, December
5, 2007, http://www.scientificamerican.com/article.cfm?id=experts-parrots-mimic.

The Chipmunk

52   *"The earliest varieties of almonds were found in China;" were brought over from Spain by the Franciscan Padres*
Nut Farm [Mike &TomGeyer],"AlmondHistory,"http://www.nutsforalmonds.com/history.htm.

52   *Good quality protein; fiber and vitamin E; "unique blend of* minerals,"
Melody Rhodes, "Eating Almonds for Good Health: Mineral-Rich Almond Nuts Good for Bone & Cardiovascular
Health," Holistic Nutrition, Suite 101.com, April 2, 2008, .
http://melodyrhodes.suite101.com/almonds-and-good-health-a49468.

Nature's Number 1 Forager

53   *"How much these cheek pouches can hold"*
Palisades Interstate Park Commission [New Jersey Section], ed., "Chipmunks Ahoy!,"
Cliff Notes, Sept / Oct 2004, http://www.njpalisades.org/cn2004_09-10.htm.

53   *Tunneling activity – an important role in the dispersion of seeds* Hinterland Who's Who, Mammal Fact Sheets:
"Chipmunk, Habitat and habits, Conservation," http://www.hww.ca/en/species/mammals/chipmunk.html.

The Monkey

54   *Daily value percentages of Vitamin C and potassium*
United States Department of Health and Human Services Centers for Disease Control and
Prevention, "Fruit of the Month: Banana," Fruits and Veggies Matter,
http://www.fruitsandveggiesmatter.gov/month/banana.html.

54   *"A good snack choice for endurance athletes"*
Sanjana Nayak, "4th Burning Question: Do Bananas Contain Fat?," Nutri-Health – Your Daily Diet Gyaan, July 30, 2008, http://nutrihealth.in/2008/07/4th-burning-question-do-bananas-contain-fat.

The Entertainer

55   *"Monkeys have developed prehensile tails"*
Tom Harris, "How Rainforests Work: All Creatures, Great and Small," HowStuffWorks.com, April 17, 2001, http://science.howstuffworks.com/conservation-issues/rainforest4.htm.

The Squirrel

56   *Originated in South America; "the soldiers both the North and the South."* Vegetarians in Paradise [Zel and Reuben Allen], "Peanuts – Whada   Ya Mean It's a Bean?" Origins, Peanuts Feed the Troops," March 2002, http://www.vegparadise.com/highestperch43.html.

56   *1890, when "a St. Louis physician"*
PeanutButterLovers.com, "Where we spread it on thick!: History," A Southern Peanut Growers nonprofit trade association, representing peanut farmers in Georgia, Alabama, Florida and Mississippi, http://peanutbutterlovers.com/pb-lovers/pb101/history/.

56   *"Three pounds of peanut butter;" "Two former U.S. Presidents,"*
PeanutButterLovers.com, Spread-worthy Facts, A Southern Peanut Growers nonprofit trade association, representing peanut farmers in Georgia, Alabama, Florida, and Mississippi, http://www.peanutbutterlovers.com/pb-lovers/pb101/facts, (with permission, August 28, 2005, updated 2012).

56   *"Peanuts came with them;" fed them to the pigs*
Virginia Carolina Peanuts, "A Short Peanut History," 2003 Virginia-Carolinas Peanut Promotions - Nashville, NC, Updated Oct 05, 2007,
http://www.aboutpeanuts.com/index.php?option=com_content&task=view&id=37&Itemid
=72.

56   *A good way to add protein to a meal or snack, plus vitamins and minerals*
Nancy Clark, "Peanut Butter: A Super Sports Food," Beginner Triathlete.com, November 14, 2004, http://www.beginnertriathlete.com/cms/article-detail.asp?articleid=332.

The Little Farmer

57   *"A good look at the next squirrel you see;" a squirrel's gnawing action is very important for his survival*
Forest Preserve District of Cook County, Illinois," "Squirrels," *Nature Bulletin,* no. 5 (March 10,1945), updated June 2012. Also available online at http://www.newton.dep.anl.gov/natbltn/001-099/nb005.htm.

57   *Are physical adaptations*
Houston Arboretum & Nature Center, "The Guided Field Experience" – School Program, Fourth Grade," (curriculum, Houston Arboretum & Nature Center, 2009).

57   *Along with forests of seed and nut bearing trees*
"The origin and development of squirrels," *World Book Multimedia Encyclopedia,* deluxe ed., CD-ROM, World Book, Inc., 1999, s.v. "squirrel," (contributor: Peter D. Weigl, *Ph.D.,*
Prof. of Biology, Wake forest Univ.).

57   *"Good memory and keen sense of smell"*
"The life of squirrels," *World Book Multimedia Encyclopedia,* deluxe ed., CD-ROM, World Book, Inc., 1999, s.v. "squirrel," (contributor: Peter D. Weigl, *Ph.D.,*
Prof. of Biology, Wake forest Univ.).

Spunky Monkey

58 *"Contain hefty quantities of natural antioxidants called flavonoids"*
Jim Core, "In Chocolate, More Cocoa Means Higher Antioxidant Capacity," United States Department of Agriculture, Agriculture Research Service, April 4, 2005, http://www.ars.usda.gov/is/pr/2005/050404.2.htm?pf=1.

58 *Similar flavonoids can be found in*
Cleveland Clinic, Heart and Vascular Health & Prevention, "The Sweet Truth About Chocolate and Your Heart: What are Flavonoids?" http://my.clevelandclinic.org/heart/prevention/nutrition/chocolate.aspx (accessed August 6, 2011).

58 *"Just 1/4 ounce or 30 calories a day"*
Elana Zimelman, R.D., L.D., C.D.E., "Dark Chocolate Please," *Cooper Clinic Nutrition: Wellness Insider Lifestyle E-Newsletter*, (February 16, 2010), available on line at http://www.cooperaerobics.com/Newsletters/Wellness-Insider/2010/February-16/Print-Newsletter.aspx.

58 *"Pollinated by tiny flies called midges;" "about seven milk chocolate bars or two dark chocolate bars;"*
California Academy of Sciences, "Chocolate: The Exhibition," in association with The Field Museum, Chicago, 2005, Published in conjunction with the exhibition "Chocolate: The Exhibition," shown nationally, http://www.calacademy.org/exhibits/chocolate/chocolate.php.

58 *Have symbiotic relationships with understory trees; the bitter taste of the seeds*
Field Museum, "Chocolate and its Environment," Reference Material 9, copyright 2002 by the Field Museum, available on line at http://archive.fieldmuseum.org/chocolate/education_pdf/choc_environ_reference.pdf.

58 *"A tiny fly no bigger than the head of a pin;"*
Allen Young, curator of zoology, and vice president of collections, research, and public programs at the Milwaukee Public Museum, "No More Chocolate? How the Rain Forest and a Tiny Fly Make Chocolate Happen: The Chocolate Tree," *BioBulletin* (American Museum of Natural History), Fall 1999, http://www.amnh.org/sciencebulletins/biobulletin/biobulletin/story720.html.

59 *"Complicated in design"*
"No More Chocolate? How the Rain Forest and a Tiny Fly Make Chocolate Happen: The Chocolate Tree," *BioBulletin* (American Museum of Natural History), Fall 1999, http://www.amnh.org/sciencebulletins/biobulletin/biobulletin/story721.html.

Chapter 5 – It␣s a Green Thing

62 *"A sense of wonder and joy in nature"*
Richard Louv, *Last Child in the Woods* (Chapel Hill, NC: Algonquin Books, 2005), 221.

63 *Less time for "homework, exercising or exploring"*
Emily Listfield, "Born to be Wired," *Houston Chronicle: Parade*, (October 9, 2011), 14.

Stump the Naturalist - Part 1

71 *Most important **bird** pollinator of wildflowers*
United States Forest Service, Celebrating Wildflowers: Bird Pollination," "http://www.fs.fed.us/wildflowers/pollinators/animals/birds.shtml.

71 *The chicken or the egg*
Rudolph L. Schreiber, Antony W. Diamond, Roger Tony Peterson, Walter Cronkite, "Save the Birds," For the world of tomorrow, A PRO NATURE book, First American Edition (Boston, Massachusetts: Houghton Mifflin Company,1989), 2.

71   *Polar bear listed as threatened*
Joe Pouliot, "U.S. Government Affirms that Climate Change is Putting Polar Bears in Peril,"
(press release, World Wildlife Fund, May 14,2008),
http://www.worldwildlife.org/who/media/press/2008/WWFPresitem9010.html.

Stump the Naturalist – Part 2

75   *Carnivorous plants like the Venus Fly Trap*
Carl Zimmer, "Fatal Attraction: They lure insects into death traps, then gorge on their flesh. Is that any way for a
plant to behave?" *National Geographic*, March 2010, Also available online at
http://ngm.nationalgeographic.com/2010/03/carnivorous-plants/zimmer-text,
(accessed April 4, 2010).

Wildlife Birthday Party

77   *Lead children on a scavenger hunt*
With permission: "Forest Detective Scavenger Hunt, " (curriculum, and birthday parties, Houston Arboretum &
Nature Center). Programs and activities can be accessed on line at:
www.houstonarboretum.org.

Chapter 6 – Recipes for Vibrant Living

98   *Health care went beyond just medicine*
Consulate General of Switzerland, "Swiss Recipe: Birchermuesli, Swiss Roots USA:
Heritage,
http://swissroots.headwire.com/swissroots/en/stories/heritage/Heritage/Swiss%20Recipes/
Birchermuesli (accessed August 11, 2011).

102 *They have also been linked to eye and brain health*
On eye health:
MayoClinic.com, Dry Macular Degeneration: Prevention, "Include fish in your diet,"(Mayo Clinic staff, November
20, 2012), http://www.mayoclinic.com/health/macular-
degeneration/DS00284/DSECTION=prevention.

102 On brain health:
NBC Nightly News, New York, NY: NBC Universal, "Fish Oil Linked to Brain Health, "
Bryan Williams/Dr. Nancy Snyderman reporting, February 27, 2012,
Video available on line at
http://www.nbcnews.com/video/nightly-news/46548774#46548774.